The Illustrated Guide to Assistive Technology and Devices

The Illustrated Guide to Assistive Technology and Devices

Tools and Gadgets for Living Independently

Suzanne Robitaille

demos
HEALTH
New York

Visit our web site at www.demosmedpub.com

Medical information provided by Demos Health, in the absence of a visit with a healthcare professional, must be considered as an educational service only. This book is not designed to replace a physician's independent judgment about the appropriateness or risks of a procedure or therapy for a given patient. Our purpose is to provide you with information that will help you make your own healthcare decisions.

The information and opinions provided here are believed to be accurate and sound, based on the best judgment available to the authors, editors, and publisher, but readers who fail to consult appropriate health authorities assume the risk of any injuries. The publisher is not responsible for errors or omissions. The editors and publisher welcome any reader to report to the publisher any discrepancies or inaccuracies noticed.

Library of Congress Cataloging-in-Publication Data

Robitaille, Suzanne.
    The illustrated guide to assistive technology and devices: tools and gadgets for living independently / Suzanne Robitaille.
       p. cm.
    Includes index.
    ISBN 978–1–932603–80–4
    1. Self-help devices for people with disabilities—United States. 2. Computerized self-help devices for people with disabilities—United States. 3. Communication devices for people with disabilities—United States. 4. People with disabilities—Rehabilitation—United States. I. Title.

HV1569.5.R63 2010
681'.761—dc22   2009036181

Special discounts on bulk quantities of Demos Health books are available to corporations, professional associations, pharmaceutical companies, health care organizations, and other qualifying groups. For details, please contact:

Special Sales Department
Demos Medical Publishing
11 W. 42nd Street, 15th Floor
New York, NY 10036
Phone: 800–532–8663 or 212–683–0072
Fax: 212–941–7842
E-mail: rsantana@demosmedpub.com

Made in the United States of America
09 10 11 12   5 4 3 2 1

To Gregory, for teaching me to soar

Contents

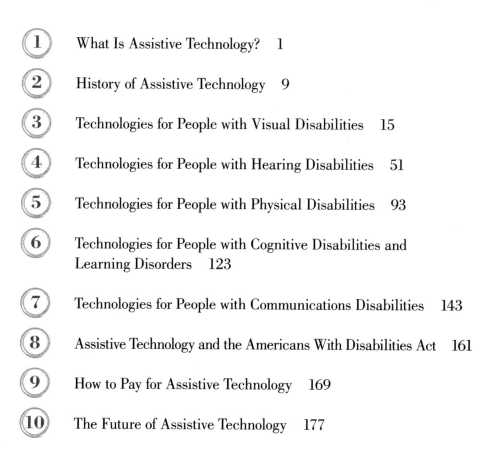

Foreword

Imagine you're starting to lose your vision—something that happens to many of us as we grow older. Suddenly the magazines and newspapers you're used to reading every day are no longer available to you. The books you enjoy are gone. Even more importantly, you may not be able to continue working if you cannot read the documents and manuals you need for your job. If you are young and a student, how do you read your textbooks and class assignments? The challenge of learning takes on a whole new meaning for you.

Twenty years ago, people with vision problems needed to spend more than $5,000 to get a computer that talked, along with a scanner that made textbooks and other publications accessible. Thankfully, today there are more options—and the situation is getting better. Manufacturers are building assistive technologies directly into their computers, making them more accessible to people with disabilities. Apple's and Microsoft's latest operating systems have free, built-in screen readers, which are speech engines that read aloud words on a screen for the blind and visually impaired. There is also a free, open source screen reader available for download, funded by Mozilla, Microsoft, Yahoo!, Adobe, and other tech giants, which will expand access to information for those who need it most.

Today, user-friendly, inexpensive mobile technology offers an unprecedented opportunity to reach even the most disadvantaged communities. This is the future of assistive technology: affordable devices and gadgets that are universally designed and accessible to everyone, including people with disabilities. Imagine a cell phone that will see for those who cannot see, listen for those who cannot hear, speak for those who cannot speak, remember for those who cannot remember, translate for those who do not understand, and guide those who are lost.

I have been working in the field of assistive technology for more than two decades. I entered the field by chance. As a student at the California Institute of Technology in the 1970s, I had planned to become an astronaut. This all changed during a modern optics class, in which I learned how to develop pattern recognition systems. In class we learned how to build a smart bomb with a camera in the nose, which used optical pattern recognition to find a target in the distance and blow it up. I left the class knowing that there had to be a way to use this technology to help rather than hurt people.

My idea was to use optical pattern recognition to build the world's first affordable reading machine for the blind. It was a few more years before I started my deliberately nonprofit company, Arkenstone, to begin to produce this device. Our first prototype, built in 1987, cost almost $50,000. It took a page of text and ran it through a scanner, taking a digital photograph of the page. The optical character recognition software turned the picture of the page into a word-processor text file, just as if someone had typed it in by hand. Then a voice synthesizer read the text aloud in a very mechanical voice.

We anticipated that the market for this machine would be $1 million per year, but within three years our nonprofit social enterprise was making five times that revenue annually. By 2000, we had provided more than 35,000 reading systems in sixty countries that could read in a dozen languages.

How were we able to do this? Simple. As the technology components became cheaper, more blind people were able to afford the machine. Over ten years the cost of an Arkenstone reading system dropped from $5,000 to $1,200. Each time the price went down, our unit volumes went up—and more people got the benefit of this technology.

We also discovered that nearly 20 percent of our users were not blind but dyslexic. The original software highlighted each word as it was spoken, making it an ideal reading tool for users with dyslexia and other learning disabilities.

In 2000, we renamed our nonprofit company Benetech, which stands for "beneficial technology." Benetech is a collection of social enterprises, hybrids that combine the best aspects of business skills and nonprofit heart to create innovative solutions to the problems facing humanity. One of our objectives is to empower the world's 650 million people with disabilities through technology.

This is essential. Technology touches every part of our lives, from education and work to entertainment and shopping. If we don't make technology accessible to everyone—including people with disabilities—we may find someone we love, or even ourselves, left behind. And to remain globally competitive, we must ensure that all of our citizens have the tools they need to participate independently in school and in the workplace.

One of Benetech's biggest initiatives, Bookshare, was inspired by my then 14-year-old son Jimmy, who introduced me to Napster, the music-sharing Web site. I quickly recognized how a Napster-style approach could help people with disabilities. Hundreds of Arkenstone users were independently scanning the exact same books. What if they could share scanned books over the Internet? It would save many, many hours of effort and greatly increase the availability of books.

Today Bookshare is a digital library with more than 60,000 titles, built initially by people with vision, learning, and physical disabilities who volunteered to scan books into digital formats and upload them to the Bookshare Web site. More than 35 publishers have partnered with Bookshare to upload their digital files directly to our library so that our members have access to an enormous variety of books, including the majority of titles on the *New York Times* bestseller list and reference books such as *Encyclopaedia Britannica*. Once downloaded, these digital books can be read aloud using synthesized speech, enlarged for those with low vision, or rendered in electronic print or braille.

In 2007, the U.S. Department of Education awarded Bookshare a five-year contract to deliver accessible books free to all qualified K–12 students with print disabilities in the United States. Bookshare is a great example of how social enterprise (i.e., government, charity, and business working together) can devise a much-needed solution to a pressing concern.

Indeed, the U.S. government, by passing laws such as the Americans with Disabilities Act, the Tech Act, and the Individuals with Disabilities Education Act, helps to get assistive technologies into the hands of the people who need them. Private insurance helps, too, but only for some people and some technologies.

At Benetech, we imagine a world where everyone on the planet has access to the assistive technologies that he or she needs for employment, education, and social inclusion. The reality is that we're not there yet because of the high costs associated with building specialized devices and the training and support associated with them.

If all mainstream technology companies design accessibility into their products from the beginning, those with disabilities won't be left behind. The market for assistive technology will actually strengthen in response: with basic technologies taken care of, people with disabilities will thrive economically, and the market for premium assistive technologies will expand as this group can afford newer and better solutions (and costs will go down, too).

We're already seeing this happen with the nation's 75 million baby boomers, many of whom are purchasing home appliances and other gadgets that are geared to their age-related disabilities, such as arthritis and macular degeneration.

I firmly believe that technology can be an immense force for good in the world. But I've also learned that this won't happen in a vacuum. We in the technology industry must work together to create more accessible products at prices that people can afford. Governments must actively seek private and public sector solutions, and social enterprises should play a larger role in effecting change.

Ultimately, it's about ensuring access to the tools people with disabilities need to pursue their dreams of independence. We have the technology; we just need to raise the floor for everyone.

Every person with a disability should have the basic tools he or she needs to ensure equal access to information and knowledge.

And we should also educate—through books such as *The Illustrated Guide to Assistive Technology and Devices*—to help people with disabilities find what they need to take charge of their lives. All of these efforts will deliver sustainable change and, ideally, enable each person on the planet to access the information he or she needs for education, employment, health, and social inclusion.

Jim Fruchterman
Founder and CEO of Benetech
Palo Alto, California

| Preface

If we all did the things we are capable of doing, we would literally astound ourselves.

—Thomas A. Edison

I never quite understood why most assistive technology books were relegated to obscure sections in national bookstore chains. Assistive technology is a topic that's as worthy as any management, human resource, and corporate responsibility title on today's business bookrack, or any mainstream health book at the front of the store,

I'm a business writer at heart, having worked for BusinessWeek.com as an assistive technology writer. I'm naturally interested in technologies that will help improve the working life of a person with a disability, as well as better their daily living needs. In March 2009, I founded a blog and Web site, Abledbody.com (www.abledbody.com), which covers assistive technology and disability news for people with disabilities.

So I'm writing this book about assistive technology in a way that has not been done before. I wish to help people with disabilities make informed purchasing decisions that will help them to succeed in their workplace and lifespace. At the same time I want to teach others, including family members, educators, and employers, how individual technologies are able to make an impact on a disabled person's life and open their opportunities for advancement and prosperity.

This book isn't going to focus on just *any* technology for *anyone* with a disability. I simply don't have that kind of expertise (or the wherewithal). I won't focus on educational or rehabilitative technologies. I'll leave that to the educators and medical professionals. Rather, I'll draw on my own experience living with a disability and working in several Fortune 500 companies where I found that any device or gadget that I needed I had to find on my own.

Aside from professional and personal experience, I interviewed a lot of people before sitting down to pen these chapters. Jay Leventhal, formerly the editor of AccessWorld at the American Foundation of the Blind, was extremely helpful and thoughtful in helping me shape the chapters on vision loss. Paul Willington of TecEar supplied me with details around assistive listening devices for the deaf and hard of hearing. Mark Felling, president of Broadened Horizons, offered up excellent overviews of adaptive phones and other equipment for people with physical limitations. Merideth Berger, director of the Clarke School for the Deaf in New York, taught me about different technologies for note taking and meetings for people who are deaf and hearing impaired. I also want to thank my editor, Noreen Henson, for developing the idea for the book and trusting me to bring it to life; and my intern, Tess Timoshin, for helping me pull together illustrations and other resources. Of course none of this would be possible without the help of the more than 100 assistive technology vendors; their products truly inform this book and are helping millions of people with disabilities.

Most important to me when writing this book was making sure I captured the most useful and up-to-date technologies that are available for purchase today. Some of these devices, of course, are cost-prohibitive, so I am operating under a few assumptions: First, that employers who hire qualified people with disabilities will also work to provide them with reasonable accommodations, similar to how employers also provide health insurance to all of their employees regardless of any preexisting conditions. Providing accommodations is a provision of the Americans with Disabilities Act (ADA). Second, the Individuals with Disabilities Education Act (IDEA) includes provisions for assistive technologies for all students up to grade 12. Third, state agencies, under the Tech Act, provide many of the technologies that appear in this book to people with disabilities.

Finally, the reality is that it's expensive to have a disability, and to pretend that it isn't would be a lie. People with disabilities very often have to make a choice to use their income to purchase technologies that will help them live fulfilling lives. This book reflects those choices, which are difficult for many in this demographic to make.

If I can supply people with disabilities, their families, educators, and employers with a modicum of knowledge to help them make thoughtful and intelligent purchasing decisions about assistive technology, and if a person with a disability is able to use any of technologies in this book to fabricate a more independent and productive life, I will have achieved my goal.

The Illustrated Guide to Assistive Technology and Devices

What Is Assistive Technology?

1

Self-preservation is the first law of nature.
—Samuel Butler

Having a disability isn't easy. Believe me, I know. I have had a hearing disability since I was four years old. Growing up profoundly deaf impacted my education, my lifestyle, and eventually my employment. Indirectly, it affected my parents, my sister, my teachers, my friends, and my bosses.

But being deaf was also a blessing. It helped me build character; it gave me insight into a more realistic world than the one my peers lived in; and it brought for me a love of books, and of writing, which my wonderful mother—who, like the rest of my family, was hearing—encouraged me to pursue as a career.

The definition of "disability" is any physical or mental impairment that substantially limits a major life activity. Disabilities include, but are not limited to, learning disabilities, blindness or low vision, hearing loss, speech impairments, and mobility impairments. Assistive technologies have helped many people to circumvent, mitigate, or eliminate the barriers to major life activities.

In my case, I couldn't comprehend language or use the telephone with just my hearing. When I was twenty-seven I got a cochlear implant; the surgery removed my natural hearing forever and replaced it with artificial hearing. Today I can hear on the phone. I have a device implanted inside my head that's attached to a processor I wear behind my ear. I made the choice—and for me it was a good one—to allow assistive technology to play a large role in my life so that I could hear again.

When I tell people I write about assistive technology, I can see their eyes glaze over—that is, until I tell them that this is technology that helps people with disabilities succeed in the workplace and life space. Then their faces light up: "Oh my, that's so wonderful," they exclaim. "My sister has a learning disability" or "Gee, my father is losing his hearing."

Suddenly, they can relate. That's because disability affects most of us in one way or another. In the United States, 54 million people have a physical or mental disability. That's 20 percent of the population. More than 20 million families have at least one family member who has been touched by disability. And one can add to that the 80 million baby boomers, the growing number of children with special needs, and the thousands of soldiers returning from Iraq and Afghanistan who have service-connected disabilities such as limb loss and brain injury.

Today, disability has been threaded into our national discourse. It affects health care, employment, education, and recreation. It has an impact on the person's physical and financial health and well-being, not to mention the strain on a family trying to provide care and attention.

That's why technology is so important for people with disabilities. Assistive technology devices can help improve physical or mental functioning, alleviate a disorder or impairment, prevent the worsening of a condition, improve a person's capacity to learn, or even replace a missing limb.

Types of Assistive Technology

Assistive technology comes in many different shapes, sizes, and packages. It can be acquired commercially off the shelf, modified or customized, or designed specifically for one or more disability types. The one thing that all assistive technologies have in common is that it's a capability enhancer.

There are ten classes of assistive technology devices, categorized by their main objective:

1. Architectural elements, such as adaptations to the home and other premises
2. Sensory elements, such as aids for communication and hearing
3. Computers, such as software and hardware
4. Controls, including environmental controls
5. Aids for independent living, such as personal care items
6. Prostheses and orthoses

7. Aids for personal mobility, including wheelchairs
8. Modified furniture and furnishings
9. Aids for recreation and sports
10. Services, such as device selection and training

This classification is widely used in the U.S. and around the world.

In addition, assistive technology can be "no-tech," such as Velcro for fastening your shirt; "low-tech," such as a walking cane; or "high-tech," such as screen-reading software. It can be specially designed equipment for the disabled or standard equipment that has been modified for their use. Here are some more examples:

- Hearing aids
- Access ramps
- Wheelchairs
- Speech generators
- Talking books
- Closed-captioned television

In this book I discuss all types of assistive technology, looking at technologies that can aid individuals in their work, home, and lifestyle. These devices include the various types of low-tech and high-tech hardware, software, and gadgets that are available to people with different disabilities. However, I will pay closer attention to products on the higher end of the technology spectrum.

For example, people with limited hand function may use a keyboard with large keys or a special mouse to operate a computer, people who are blind may use software that reads text on the screen in a computer-generated voice, people with low vision may use software that enlarges screen content, people who are deaf may use a text telephone (TTY), and people with speech impairments may use a device that speaks out loud as they enter text via a keyboard.

In many cases, higher-tech assistive technology is more expensive, is harder to find, and has a learning curve, but the results can be extraordinary, in the sense that these are life-changing devices. Without these technologies, someone might not be able to go to school, sustain a job, or communicate with family members.

Defining Assistive Technology

Many people in my field don't like the term "assistive technology." It's medical sounding, doesn't trip off the tongue, and, quite frankly, sounds boring. The legal definition of assistive technology was first published in the Technology-Related Assistance for Individuals with Disabilities Act of 1988, known today as the Tech Act. This act was replaced with the Assistive Technology Act of 1998, which established a grant program to provide states with funding for assistive technology products and services. In 2004 the law was amended to mandate, in some instances, that states provide alternative financing and loans for assistive technologies. I talk more about this in Chapter 9, "How to Pay for Assistive Technology."

Congress defines assistive technology in Section 3 of the 1998 Tech Act as follows:

> Assistive technology is any item, piece of equipment, or product system, whether acquired commercially or off the shelf, modified or customized, that is used to increase, maintain, or improve the functional capabilities of a person with a disability.

People with disabilities might be pleased or even surprised about what the U.S. government has to say on assistive technology and disability. According to the Assistive Technology Act, disability is "a natural part of the human experience and in no way diminishes the right of individuals to live independently, enjoy self-determination and make choices, benefit from an education, pursue meaningful careers, and enjoy full inclusion and integration in the economic, political, social, cultural, and educational mainstream of society in the United States."

Under the Assistive Technology Act, the Department of Education provides grants and funding to increase the "availability [of] and access to assistive technology devices and services" that will "significantly benefit individuals with disabilities of all ages." Keep in mind that this law was passed two years before the proliferation of mobile devices, smartphones, mp3 players, and electronic book readers. It also preceded the Americans with Disabilities Act (1990)—the landmark civil rights legislation for people with disabilities—which I'll talk about later in this book.

On a less formal note, a former BusinessWeek.com colleague, John Williams, should get some credit for coining the phrase "assistive technology." John has been writing about disability and assistive technology since 1980—a decade before the Americans with Disabilities Act was passed into law. He also started the Assistive Technology column, which I took over after he left *BusinessWeek* in 2001 and continued until the end of 2004.

Benefits of Assistive Technology

The benefits of assistive technology cross categories of age, disability, and health challenges. From young children to seniors, people may face a range of physical and cognitive limitations. Today, there are thousands of assistive technology products on the market to help people with disabilities with all sorts of needs, from the simple to the sophisticated. If you or someone you know has difficulty typing on a keyboard, reading a document, or hearing the TV, there's probably a product that will fit your needs or theirs. It's really just a matter of finding the right technology and figuring out how to use it.

Sometimes I meet people who are afraid of using assistive technology because it seems like a crutch. Believe me when I say it is not. In all the conversations I've had with people outside of the assistive technology world, they use words such as "cool," "brave," and "inspiring."

This is especially noticeable when the assistive technology is associated with helping someone who is already doing something well do it even better: like Oscar Pistorius, the Paralympic athlete from South Africa who straps on blade runners—prosthetic legs—to run 100-meter races, or Stephen Hawking, the brilliant astrophysicist with a neuromuscular disability who uses a device that helps him communicate his theories about black holes.

Users of assistive technology must acknowledge that the device exists to help them. There is no stigma in using assistive technology as a daily or occasional aid in your life. Quite honestly, self-preservation is a human responsibility; it's a hard world out there, and if you want to thrive, it is wise to do whatever it takes to stay on top of your game.

With assistive technology, the families of people with disabilities benefit too. Instead of a wife having to read the mail of a person who is blind, he can read it himself using scan-and-speak software. Instead of a child making a phone call for his mother who is deaf, she can do it herself in sign language, over the Internet.

One of the most important things to remember is that, as humans, we're all temporarily abled. At one point or another, it is likely that each of us will use some form of assistive technology. If you have a disability now, you're just starting a little sooner.

Assistive technology is a life-changer. It can help individuals with disabilities increase their independence, build their self-confidence and self-esteem, improve their quality of life, and break down barriers to education and employment. The real challenge, of course, is finding the right devices and gadgets, for the right purpose, at the right price.

History of Assistive Technology

2

> *If necessity is the mother of invention, then disability is
> its grandmother.*
>
> —Unknown

In the beginning there were bullhorns. That's what hearing-impaired people used as tools to try to hear. In the 1870s, Alexander Graham Bell, whose wife was deaf, tried to develop a device for her to hear and ended up inventing the telephone. Until Louis Braille invented braille in 1824, blind people couldn't read; it wasn't until the development of "talking" reading machines, including the one invented by Ray Kurzweil in 1975, that many people with vision impairments could have access to printed material.

The history of modern assistive technology doesn't go back very far. In fact, the people who are considered the pioneers of assistive technology are still around and working on next-generation technologies. Many consider Gregg Vanderheiden, a professor at the University of Wisconsin-Madison, to be a leader in this field. In the 1970s Vanderheiden developed Auto-Com, one of the first communications devices for people who cannot speak. Today he is working on making the World Wide Web more accessible for people with disabilities.

One of Vanderheiden's partners in this initiative is Jim Fruchterman, a long-time inventor and assistive technology entrepreneur, who wrote in a 2007 op-ed in the *Sacramento Bee*:

> At an affordable price, everybody should have access to communications technology and content to meet their personal, social, educational and employment needs. We need to raise the technology floor so that all of our citizens have at least the basic tools they need to participate in our modern society. – "Everyone deserves access to technology." Online world, Sacramento Bee, June 17, 2007.

The first eyeglasses (about AD 1000) took the form of handheld lenses. It was probably an Italian monk, scientist, or craftsman who invented head-worn eyeglasses, in about 1285. When Gutenberg invented the printing press in 1456, which made printed books accessible to more people, the evolution of eyeglasses was fully under way.

We also must recognize those who pioneered mainstream technologies such as the personal computer. Without Bill Gates and Paul Allen and their colleagues at Microsoft, or Steve Jobs and Steve Wozniak and their team at Apple, or Vincent Cerf, the father of the Internet, who committed themselves early on to making their technologies accessible to the widest audience possible, the disability community wouldn't be as well equipped as they are today.

Apple's Early Start

Speaking at the Assistive Technology Oral History Project, Alan Brightman, former head of the Apple Education Foundation, noted the following:

> At Apple we made an interesting discovery after about three years of working to make the Macintosh more accessible for people with disabilities. We thought we were about accessibility, but we realized our real purpose was to fundamentally change the experience of being disabled. When we have this technology, and assuming that we can use it, all of a sudden we have a whole new range of degrees-of-freedom and we're more independent. We could almost see people sitting up straighter in their wheelchair and almost adding inches to their self-esteem. It was a phenomenal consequence of being given this new gadget; this new technology.

Source: Assistive Technology Oral History Project, with permission.

The rise of assistive technology in the United States can be traced to the pre-computer era, particularly following the Second World War, when the great number of veterans with disabilities posed a dramatic social problem and prompted the U.S. Veterans Administration to launch a prosthetic and sensory aids program, which was followed by many initiatives that spawned modern research into rehabilitation and assistive technology.

Gradually the idea took shape that a person with a disability should aim not necessarily at bodily normality but at life normality, which inspired the first programs of vocational rehabilitation intended to help people regain access to work and productive life. The Vietnam War also increased awareness about disability civil rights. Veterans who returned home with disabilities in the mid-1970s laid the groundwork for the 1990 Americans with Disabilities Act (ADA), one of the most important pieces of civil rights legislation in American history.

The ADA extends full civil rights and equal opportunities in both the public and private sectors to people with disabilities. Specifically, the law prohibits discrimination in employment, public service, public accommodations, and telecommunications on the basis of a physical or mental disability.

An excellent movie on this topic, *Music Within* (2007), chronicles the activities of Richard Pimentel, a brilliant public speaker who returns from Vietnam severely hearing impaired and finds a new purpose lobbying on behalf of Americans with disabilities.

The disability civil rights movement had to overcome not only prejudice but also physical barriers that limited access to employment and inclusion in other aspects of daily life. Activists successfully lobbied for laws that required curb cuts, ramps, and buses with wheelchair lifts.

Crucial to the movement's success was access to information and communication through technologies such as text telephones, voice-recognition systems, voice synthesizers, screen readers, and computers.

This access in turn increased the possibility of economic and social mobility. In the 1970s and 1980s, a growing population of consumers with mobility impairments fueled demand for wheelchairs and scooters to match their active lives. At the same time, barrier-free designs brought a new aesthetic to public spaces. Curb cuts are now ubiquitous in cities and towns, but they didn't exist until people with disabilities fought for them.

Advances in computer technologies have provided important stimulation for the development of assistive technology. Today, assistive technology is a specific discipline that brings together thousands of engineers, scientists, and doctors from around the world at various conferences and research centers to pave the way for a better tomorrow.

Are we there yet? No, but the future is bright, and new technologies come out of the laboratories and onto the market every year that advance the field of assistive technology and the lives of people with disabilities.

Technologies
for People
with Visual
Disabilities

3

Live without seeing, but be what you are.
—Louis Braille

For most of us, our eyes are the lens through which we see life. But nearly 10 million Americans—and 135 million people worldwide—have a visual impairment or are blind, and millions of older Americans are experiencing vision problems as they age.

Fifty years ago, there wasn't much technology to assist people with vision impairments, other than maybe a small supply of large-text and braille books. Technological advances have changed the game. Today most of us, sighted or not, use computers almost daily, whether for working, shopping online, listening to music, or getting money out of an ATM.

The computer is both a marvel and a menace for people with vision impairments. That's because today's computers operate using a graphical user interface, or GUI, to depict information on a screen. Think of how Microsoft Word uses a variety of fonts and colors and lets users interact with icons such as a paintbrush or a clipboard.

For people with mild vision loss, there are programs that can enlarge text and icons to make computer software more usable. But a GUI isn't accessible at all for those with severe vision loss or blindness. More advanced assistive technologies are needed to maneuver through the computer system. Fortunately, many such devices and gadgets exist today, including screen readers, text-to-speech software, and braille keyboards.

In this chapter I'll first look at assistive technologies that are available for people who have any range of low vision. Then I'll discuss technologies for people who are blind.

Determining Your Degree of Vision Loss

EFPTOZLPED. Does this word mean anything to you? It's the sequence of letters used in a doctor's office chart to test clearness

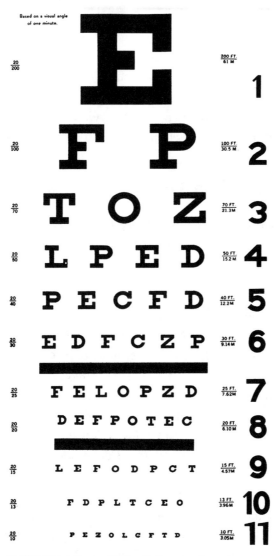

Snellen Chart. (Source: Wikimedia Commons.)

of sight from a distance, known as the Snellen chart, named after Dutch ophthalmologist Herman Snellen.

People who can read the eighth line of the chart are considered to have 20/20 vision, which is regarded as the mean, or normal, vision. Someone with 20/40 vision can see only at twenty feet what a normal person can see from forty feet. Those who can read only the first or second line of a Snellen chart are determined to have 20/400 or 20/200 vision, respectively, and probably require eyeglasses for driving and other activities. A person unable to read these letters with eyeglasses is considered legally blind.

Vision loss can occur as a result of eye disorders, disease, infection, or brain and nerve disorders. As we age, conditions such as cataracts, glaucoma, and age-related macular degeneration are more likely to affect our sight and cause low vision.

Understanding Vision

Visual impairments occur to varying degrees, though anyone with noncorrectable reduced vision is considered to be visually impaired.

- Near-normal vision refers to mild vision loss in the range 20/30 to 20/60.
- Moderate low vision refers to vision in the range 20/70 to 20/160. It is a significant reduction in sight that ordinary eyeglasses, contact lenses, or medical treatment cannot completely correct.
- Severe low vision refers to vision in the range 20/200 to 20/400. People who have 20/200 or worse vision, or a visual field of twenty degrees or less, are considered legally blind. Being legally blind marks an entry point for many low-vision services and benefits.
- Profound low vision refers to vision in the range 20/500 to 20/1,000.
- Near-total blindness refers to vision that is less than 20/1,000.
- Total blindness is considered to be present when a person has no light perception. People who are totally blind rely on nonvisual ways to absorb information and navigate the world.

Source: U.S. National Library of Medicine and the National Institutes of Health (www.nlm.nih.gov), Sept. 2009.

Assistive Technologies for Low Vision

Kathy, sixty-two, is a secretary at a sign company. Her vision has been causing her problems in the past few years. Her eyeglasses are helpful, but she still has trouble making out the words on invoices. Kathy uses a magnifier to read hard-copy invoices. She has a large, twenty-three-inch, computer monitor and has set up her screen to display larger text and icons. She also uses her computer's built-in magnification program when she needs to read documents on her screen. To make typing easier, Kathy purchased large keyboard labels that stick on top of her regular QWERTY keyboard. To add up purchase orders, Kathy uses a jumbo-sized calculator and is considering getting one that has speech capabilities.

Kathy is a baby boomer whose vision has been impaired by the effects of aging. Her generation will be the first to retire from the workforce adept in using computers to shop, upload pictures, and connect with family and friends via e-mail and video chat. For this reason, it is important that baby boomers have access to assistive technologies that will help them remain independent and productive in the workplace and in daily living.

Computer and Electronics Access

There are several types of programs that can help users with low vision to access the information on their computer screen. Some are built into the computer's operating system (OS). This is the best place to get started.

On Microsoft's Windows (Vista and 7) accessibility features are in the Ease of Access Center in the control panel. From here you can:

- Set the screen resolution to a lower number of pixels (for example, 800 × 600), which will increase the size of the text, graphics, and other screen elements
- Turn on the cursor enlarger and Magnifier, a magnification program that lets you enlarge a portion of your computer screen in a separate window to make it easier to see

- Turn on Narrator, a basic text-to-speech program that reads what is displayed on your screen
- Adjust the size of the icons and font color or background contrasts as needed
- Take an optional questionnaire to help set your preferences

The latest version of Windows, called Windows 7, has an improved Magnifier that will allow easier magnification of all onscreen information either in full-screen mode, which zooms the whole screen, or in lens mode, which zooms a particular area.

Apple's current Macintosh computers run on Mac OS X, which includes the Tiger, Leopard, and Snow Leopard versions. For accessibility options, go to System Preferences and choose the Universal Access icon. From here you can:

- In the Seeing tab, turn on the built-in screen magnifier, called Zoom, and change or enhance the contrast
- In the Mouse & Trackpad tab, turn on a cursor enlarger
- In the Seeing tab, turn on VoiceOver, Apple's proprietary screen reader, which provides spoken audio descriptions and can be controlled from the keyboard

The VoiceOver screen reader is widely used by people with vision impairments and comes with a high-quality text-to-speech voice known as Alex, as well as a variety of other male and female voices. You can even choose musically infused voices. Cello or pipe organ, anyone?

PC or Mac?

There is an ongoing debate over built-in versus separate assistive technologies for the personal computer. Apple makes its own assistive technology applications, which means that getting an upgrade is as simple as downloading it from Apple's Web site; you don't have to buy a whole new product. Microsoft, in contrast, partners with 180 vendors that make products to work with Windows and can offer more choices to the customer. Both Apple and Microsoft have demonstrated their commitment to accessibility over the years. Each has a dedicated Web site that details the company's initiatives, including Apple's work on its proprietary screen reader, VoiceOver, and Microsoft's work in making Word documents available in alternative formats for people who are blind. Go to these Web sites to read more: www.microsoft.com/enable and www.apple.com/accessibility.

Monitors

Remember Kathy, our sixty-two-year-old secretary? She was able to purchase a twenty-three-inch computer monitor for her workstation. The best monitors for low vision are ones nineteen inches or larger, because these allow for larger text and images to be displayed at a comfortable viewing distance. Larger monitors of nineteen and twenty-one inches have become more affordable.

Another option is to attach your computer to a flat-screen television that measures thirty or more inches. Low-vision users may also benefit from monitor arms that can be adjusted to move the computer screen up, down, forward, or backward. You can buy these from Access Ingenuity.

Keyboards and Mice

Keyboards and mice are among the more frustrating devices for people with low vision. In a perfect world, we'd all be able to control our computers strictly using our voice (or even our feet), but that hasn't happened yet.

For now, the best bet for people with low vision who have trouble seeing the keys on a keyboard is to purchase a high-contrast keyboard, such as a black-and-yellow combination with a bigger and bolder typeface that helps the keys stand out. Another option is a set of large-print or high-contrast keyboard labels that you stick on top of your keyboard. Of course, if you use a laptop you can attach any type of assistive keyboard using a USB port.

Note-Taking Devices

Greg is a vice president at a financial services company. He has low vision. Greg attends a lot of meetings but would prefer to take notes orally rather than in writing. Greg uses a digital voice recorder during meetings, which is passed around to whoever is speaking. Later, Greg types up notes on his computer and prints them in large text. Sometimes, if it's not too distracting for the other participants, Greg brings his laptop to meetings and types notes. He later uses a speech synthesizer that read his notes aloud to him so he can make corrections.

People who are blind or visually impaired long relied on cassettes to make voice recordings of meetings, class lectures, and other situations where they wanted auditory access to information. However, cassette recorders were expensive and cumbersome, and the recordings had to be played from beginning to end.

Digital voice recorders have made things easier. Today's recorders are affordable and extremely portable, and one device can hold lots of information. Many digital voice recorders on the market also allow bookmarks to be inserted into a recording so that specific parts can be located easily for later review. Both Access Ingenuity and the American Printing House for the Blind sell such recorders.

Dedicated Word Processors

Another method of taking notes, which may appeal to older people with vision loss who don't need all the bells and whistles

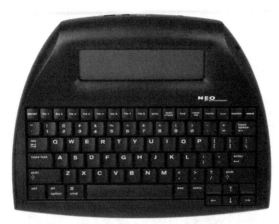

NEO Word Processor. *The AlphaSmart NEO word processor can be used for writing and note taking. (Source: Printed with permission from Renaissance Learning, Inc.)*

of a personal computer, is a dedicated word processor. These devices usually consist of a QWERTY keyboard and a small, four- to eight-line text display. This display is usually too small to be read by people with low vision, but the information can be saved as an electronic file and transferred to a computer to be spoken aloud. The NEO by AlphaSmart/Renaissance Learning, and the Dana, its Palm OS–powered counterpart, are two good choices.

Talking Word Processors

On a standard computer or laptop, you can also use software that provides auditory feedback as you type. Don Johnston's Write:OutLoud is a talking word processor and writing software program aimed at students. You can also turn on the text-to-speech engine on your computer and use it in word-processing programs such as Notepad on a Windows computer and TextEdit on a Mac.

Netbooks

If you have basic to intermediate computer and word-processing skills, you may want to consider a netbook—the latest trend in

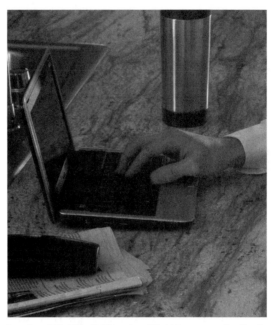

Inspiron Mini. *The Dell Inspiron Mini 9 is a compact netbook weighing less than three pounds. (Source: Photo courtesy of Dell Inc.)*

personal computing. Netbooks are very small, light, and portable laptop computers designed for wireless communication and browsing the Internet.

Most netbooks run on the Windows operating system and include the popular Microsoft Word software. Models include the Dell Inspiron Mini, HP Mini 1000, and Lenovo IdeaPad. Netbooks cost $300 on average, which makes them less expensive than a personal computer. Preferences can also be adjusted for accessibility, such as font size, though the screens are only about ten inches in size.

TIP *Dedicated word processors and netbooks are beneficial for users with low vision. Those who have more serious visual impairments or are blind should consider accessible personal digital assistants (PDAs), which are discussed in the blindness section.*

Cell Phones

You can buy a cell phone from Code Factory with a screen magnifier called Mobile Magnifier, which works with the Symbian and Windows Mobile operating platforms. (Nokia phones and some Motorola phones run on the Symbian platform.) Mobile Magnifier offers ten levels of enlargement for screen contents, with a variety of color schemes and contrasts. Nuance makes a similar magnification device for Symbian-based phones called Nuance ZOOMS.

TIP *If you're an AT&T customer, AT&T will provide Mobile Magnifier on an AT&T phone for $89 as of this book's publication date.*

Print Access

One of the biggest frustrations by far for people with vision impairments is trying to find large-print books at the local bookstore or library. While they do exist, it's like looking for a needle in a haystack.

If you're not a technophobe, consider downloading audiobooks from Apple's iTunes store, Amazon.com, or Audible.com and listening to them on your favorite mp3 player, such as an iPod. This takes the hassle out of trying to find, purchase or borrow, and read a large-print book.

For those who still prefer to snuggle up with a good book, there are a variety of options. New on the market are electronic readers that can read a book out loud, with no other equipment necessary. ABISee makes the Eye-Pal SOLO, a motion-activated device that reads aloud text from any book or printed material. It can also be connected to a computer or TV monitor and can highlight the words as it speaks them.

Another good option is an e-book reader such as the Kindle from Amazon or Sony's Reader. These slim, lightweight devices allow you to purchase and download books and periodicals from a Web site or wirelessly, using Bluetooth technology, and read them at your leisure. The font and text sizes can be adjusted for low-vision readers, and unlike reading on a computer screen, an e-book reader screen looks like real paper and displays clear text and crisp images. As of now, e-book readers cost $300 and upward, but more technology providers are releasing newer and less expensive versions.

Electronic Magnifiers

If Sherlock Holmes had had an electronic magnifier, he might have solved those crime mysteries much more quickly. Electronic magnifiers use video cameras to offer a higher degree and wider range of magnification than can be achieved practically with a traditional magnifier.

Electronic magnifiers are designed for people who have low vision who need to view a variety of materials, including small type (such as the nutrition label on a can), printed or handwritten text, and graphical materials such as photographs and maps. They're particularly useful for students and for employees who don't work in a traditional office environment, such as artists or historians. Some models offer advanced options such as reverse polarity (light text on a dark background) and the ability to function under a wider variety of lighting conditions.

Most of the major manufacturers of electronic magnifiers make models that are computer compatible; so just one monitor is needed, and you can switch between the computer and the electronic magnifier. Some systems are even laptop compatible.

While desktop models offer the greatest variety, there are also portable models on the market, including the kind that can be mounted on the head. These can be used for distance viewing of sporting events, lectures, and concerts.

Less expensive are pocket magnifiers, which are sometimes marketed toward older people with low vision to help them write checks, read books, and do crossword puzzles and needlepoint. They serve as a quick fix for those who want to carry a small device in their pocket to read, say, a restaurant menu. But pocket

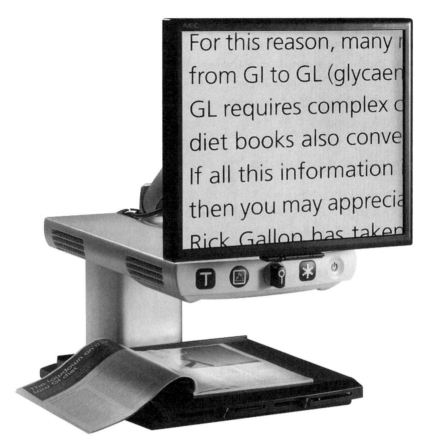

SmartView Xtend. *The SmartView Xtend from HumanWare is a desktop magnifier for low vision loss. (Source: Photo courtesy of HumanWare USA.)*

models can't be used to read as wide a range of materials as their desktop counterparts.

HumanWare makes the SmartView Xtend, a desktop model, and the SmartView Graduate, a portable model. Freedom Scientific makes a desktop model called the TOPAZ and a handheld video magnifier called the OPAL. Also, Optelec makes the FarView—a portable magnifier that the company says is "designed for an active lifestyle."

Digital Imaging Systems

Even more sophisticated are digital imaging systems, or auto readers. These devices look like electronic magnifiers but are much more powerful and easier to use. They work by taking a picture of a page using a digital camera and then rearranging the text onscreen. You choose how you prefer the text to appear. Some models can read the text out loud using synthesized speech. HumanWare's myReader2 lets you store up to ten pages at a time, making it easier to read and view books, magazines, maps, and photographs.

Specialized Scanning Systems

Some high-tech tools allow the user to convert printed information into multiple accessible formats, such as speech, large print, and audio. This involves either an optical scanner or optical character recognition (OCR) software. The best of both worlds combines imaging and OCR software in what are known as specialized scanning systems.

Specialized scanning systems display an exact image of a page on a computer screen (using a scanner) while running OCR software that speaks the text without altering the image. This dual approach gives a learning boost to users: hearing the speech decreases the effort required to identify visually each word being read, while seeing each word highlighted onscreen decreases the effort required to hear and understand every word spoken by the speech synthesizer, which often makes mistakes.

ABISee makes the Zoom-Ex, a combination scanner and OCR system that's small enough to fold up and fit into your laptop bag.

Imaging and OCR software, as well as specialized scanning systems, also provides comprehensive reading solutions for people who are blind, which I'll discuss in detail in the blindness section.

Handheld Magnifiers

We're used to being wired at work. Companies know that giving us a personal computer improves our productivity and allows information to be connected across networks. But at home you might be more interested in watching television or making a meal. People with low vision can still enjoy these activities with the help of simple assistive technologies.

One device that is often underused is the good old-fashioned magnifier. At restaurants across the country, I see older couples squinting to see their menus, and even borrowing each other's reading glasses. A simple magnifier lets you read any print at one-and-a-half to thirty times the original size.

There are two types of magnifiers—illuminated and nonilluminated—and there are handheld (or pocket) and stand models. Illuminated models offer several choices of lighting, including incandescent, xenon, krypton, and light-emitting diode (LED). One popular choice is the Optelec PowerMag, which comes in a variety of models. Bausch & Lomb also makes a line of round or rectangular and illuminated magnifiers.

Glare-Control Eyewear

Another problem that people with low vision experience is glare from bright light that affects their vision. For glare control, there are many types of polarized lenses that can be worn alone or on top of eyeglasses, such as those made by JP EyeWear. You may have seen people wearing such products: most look like sunglasses that cover the entire eye area, aviator style. This type of eyewear prevents light from entering from the side, reducing bounce-back from the inside of the lens while providing protection from ultraviolet light to help prevent cataracts. These lenses are ideal for driving and for any general outdoor activity where glare is present.

Large-Print/Large-Button Alternatives

Enjoying your favorite pastime doesn't have to be restricted by your vision impairment. In fact, there are many companies that specialize in making versions of their mainstream products available for those with low vision. For example, you can buy large-print playing cards and jumbo dice, large-print crossword puzzles and game books, large-print bingo cards, and large-print magazines.

If you like to sew, there are dozens of options for easy-thread needles. For controlling a television, you can buy an extra-large remote control, and many telephones also come with jumbo-sized buttons for easier navigation. Many such products can be purchased at www.shoplowvision.com.

Keen chefs should check out OXO's line of products for people with low vision, including large-print measuring cups and spoons. There are also electronic and talking timers so you won't burn that pot roast. One smart product on the market is a talking microwave oven from Hamilton Beach, which is equipped with a voice that talks you through all the operating functions and a rotary knob to enter numbers.

Appliance manufacturers such as GE, Whirlpool, Maytag, and Sears Kenmore have been working to make their products more accessible to older Americans, including those with vision impairments. This is in response to people who are blind and vision impaired complaining that they can't see digital controls well enough to use them.

For example, GE's Monogram line includes a double-wall oven with large rotary knobs and subtle clicks to measure off temperatures in twenty-five-degree increments. Whirlpool makes a washing machine and dryer line called Duet that offers easy-to-feel knobs and a distinct pointer, as well as tones that identify your cycle and speed choice. This line is widely regarded as an accessible choice.

Some manufacturers do better than others, depending on the product, so it's best to do research. *AccessWorld*, a free online publication for the blind and visually impaired, publishes periodic reviews of kitchen and other home appliances. And, of course, do check these products out for yourself; everybody's needs are different, and it's only by testing and trying out low-vision products that you'll be able to design a work or home environment that's most comfortable for you.

Blindness

Alexia, twenty-seven, is an editor for a music magazine. She is totally blind. She uses an accessible personal digital assistant with built-in speech that runs on Windows Mobile and gives her access to essential applications such as Word and Internet Explorer. Alexia uses her PDA to keep track of her daily schedule, update her contact list, send and receive e-mail, take notes, record interviews with bands and musicians, and, of course, listen to her favorite music.

Alexia isn't using a typical PDA. She's using a highly specialized device made specifically for people who are blind. In fact, most assistive technologies for blindness are nonvisual products. That means they're equipped with either braille or speech output. These products have smaller market share and a sophisticated system, which makes them far more expensive than off-the-shelf devices. It also takes longer to learn how to use them.

The good news is that the assistive technologies that have come onto the market for people who are blind are indeed life changing. Many of these products have come into existence since the advent of the personal computer—during the past thirty or so years—and have brought enhanced opportunities to people who are blind in school, at work, and in their daily lives.

If you're young enough not to remember a time when there wasn't a computer in every classroom, at every workstation, and in every living room, you may take many of these assistive devices for granted. Those who are over the age of thirty, however, are ecstatic that computers have replaced pen and paper (or braille slate and stylus), and they have an attitude of determination and perseverance when it comes to learning to use these newfangled devices and gadgets.

Technologies for Blindness

Bud, fifty-five, is a director at a nonprofit in Washington, DC, that promotes environmental responsibility. He is totally blind. He uses a computer that's equipped with a screen reader that reads aloud information displayed on his monitor. The screen reader helps him navigate his e-mail and word-processing programs and browse the Internet. Bud also uses a PDA, except his is equipped with a refreshable braille display, because he can read and write braille.

By far the most important technology for the workplace in the twenty-first century is the computer. As I discussed earlier in this chapter, however, a graphical user interface isn't ideal for a person who cannot rely on a mouse or other pointing device for access to information and communication.

To that end, there are a variety of assistive technology hardware and software devices that serve as workarounds for Alexia, Bud, and others who are blind to enable them to prepare documents, send and receive e-mail, and browse the Internet.

Screen Readers

The most sophisticated piece of technology to help computer users who are blind navigate GUIs is a screen reader. A screen reader is a software program that converts the text on the screen into speech. The program is capable of voicing all of the text displayed on the screen, including menus, dialog boxes, controls, and buttons that you can control with your keyboard.

Screen readers help users who are blind to read e-mail, surf the Web, work with word-processing applications, and perform other computer tasks. Nevertheless, screen readers aren't perfect; they make mistakes, so one common feature in screen-reading software is the ability to create a dictionary for the pronunciation of words.

For Windows-based environments, Microsoft makes a very basic screen reader called the Narrator, but for more advanced functions, screen-reader software must be bought separately. Two popular commercial screen readers are JAWS from Freedom Scientific and Window-Eyes from GW Micro.

As I mentioned earlier in this chapter, Apple makes its own very good screen reader called VoiceOver, which comes free when you buy a Macintosh computer. Alex, the new voice of Mac OS X Leopard, uses advanced Apple technologies to deliver natural intonation at extraordinarily fast speaking rates. You can even hear Alex breathe!

Darrell Shandrow, editor of the *Blind Access Journal* blog, tipped me off to two alternative screen readers that can be used in the workplace for e-mail, Web access, and word processing: System Access by Serotek and NonVisual Desktop Access (NVDA) by NV Access, which is free.

 TIP *You can customize your VoiceOver preferences and take them with you: Connect a USB flash drive to your Mac and choose Create Portable Preferences from the File menu in the VoiceOver utility.*

The Internet

A screen reader can also help someone who is blind surf the Web. Unfortunately, although the major Internet browsers, such as Internet Explorer and Safari, are accessible, many Web sites are designed in a way that some of the information is not accessible to people using screen-reading software.

The World Wide Web Consortium has established accessibility guidelines for Web designers. Interest in this topic continues to pick up steam, as many major corporations have found themselves in hot water—or facing a lawsuit—for not making their sites fully accessible.

For example, in 2007 the National Federation of the Blind sued Target Corporation for failing to make its online retail site accessible. Target agreed to pay $6 million in damages and had to hire designers to revamp its site.

A Costly Gamble

In summer [2008], Apple found itself in a pickle with the disability community. The state of Massachusetts was threatening to sue Apple for failing to make its iTunes media library accessible to blind students. Apple agreed to pay $250,000 and added audio to almost its entire iTunes library. It also decided to include audio in its latest iPod Shuffle, released this month [March 2009], which it has marketed as an accessible iPod.

Apple avoided a costly lawsuit, but other companies haven't been as fortunate. In the state of Washington, movie theater chains are being sued for failing to make closed-captioned movies available more frequently to the deaf and hard-of-hearing. This latest class-action suit has the potential to spill over into other areas of digital media, such as news streaming, TV show streaming, and movie downloads via the Internet.

Time and time again, companies spend heavily on product development and marketing, but fail to consider people with disabilities who might use their products. This oversight seems irresponsible: In the United States, 54 million adults—or one in five Americans—have a physical or mental disability. People with disabilities have a combined income of more than a trillion dollars—and are willing to spend it on products and technologies that make their lives more productive.

Brands that ignore the needs of this group relinquish an opportunity to reach this growing demographic. They also put their business at a higher risk for costly lawsuits, such as the $6 million in damages that Target paid in 2008 for failing to make some of its Web content accessible to blind people.

One way for companies to approach accessibility is to consider the principles of universal design, which requires that a product be built for everyone, including those with disabilities. For example, GE recently designed a kitchen with appliances such as a motorized adjustable sink that can be used by both tall and short people, including those in a wheelchair or those with a stature disability. GE markets the kitchen as "Real Life Design."

If universal design isn't an option, brands should consider partnering with an assistive technology provider to help configure their product to the needs of people with disabilities. Amazon, for example, recently partnered with Nuance Communications, a maker of speech-recognition technology, to add audio to its Kindle 2 electronic book reader. Companies that have an online presence should also check the latest accessibility guidelines from the World Wide Web Consortium, or W3C.

At the very least, companies should begin to think about every single consumer who might use their products at some point—including people with disabilities. Accessibility helps create more useful products, protects against lawsuits and opens doors to a new market that has been underserved for too long. Accessibility is a reality that companies can no longer afford to ignore.

Source: Reprinted with permission from Marketing Daily and Abledbody.com (March 27, 2009).

Keyboard Commands

Screen readers offer the best technology for helping a blind user navigate the menus and controls of a computer, but there's still the issue of using a mouse. Mice and other pointing devices are inaccessible to the blind and visually impaired, and while attempts have been made to devise mice and pointing devices that offer tactile feedback, they have had limited success.

Instead, users who are blind revert to using their keyboard. Most commonly used applications offer keyboard commands. A list of keyboard shortcuts can be found at www.allhotkeys.com or in the accessibility sections of Microsoft and Apple's Web sites.

In Mac OS X Snow Leopard, VoiceOver lets you control your computer using gestures on your Mac notebook's multitouch trackpad. The surface of the trackpad represents the active window on the computer, so you can touch the trackpad at a specific point to hear the item under your finger, drag to hear items named in turn as you move your finger, and flick with one finger to move to the next or previous item.

Refreshable Braille Displays

Many computer users who are blind rely on their screen reader for information output. However, in some situations, a refreshable braille display is a better option. This is a portable braille terminal that connects to your computer and lets you read and write braille. Some displays even have Bluetooth for wireless connectivity.

A refreshable braille display has a row of plastic pins that are raised or lowered in different combinations to represent the dots of the braille cell. They provide a single line of raised braille that can be refreshed by the user after it has been read. For example, you can use this gadget to read an onscreen Word document, one line at a time, in braille.

Refreshable braille displays require a screen reader, which drives the information from the computer to the display. Of course, you'll also need to be fluent in braille. But these devices can be beneficial in the workplace, especially if you're a frequent telephone user. For instance, having to listen to a screen reader and talk on the telephone simultaneously can be challenging, making this device a good choice for people who work in telephone call centers.

A few popular refreshable braille displays are Freedom Scientific's Focus line, HumanWare's BrailleConnect and Brailliant, and the ALVA Satellite. Displays are available with as few as

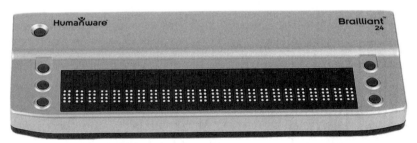

Brailliant. HumanWare's Brailliant refreshable braille display comes in several models, some of which have Bluetooth connectivity. (Source: Photo courtesy of HumanWare.)

eighteen and as many as eighty-four cells. Generally, a seventy-cell display will show one full line of onscreen text as braille; about the same number of characters across the width of a typical word processor screen.

Notetakers/Accessible PDAs

Accessible PDAs, also known as notetakers, are multitasking devices that allow you to do everything you can do on a regular PDA: word processing, surfing the Web, scheduling appointments, listening to music, storing your address list, reading e-books and synchronizing computer files.

 The advantage of a notetaker over an accessible laptop is that notetakers are a little lighter, are easier to start up, and have a longer battery life.

Notetakers operate just like regular PDAs and run on the Windows operating system. They're a little bigger than a regular PDA and look different from the ones that sighted people use. Nevertheless, these high-functioning devices have changed the way people who are blind work and interact with others, and many people say they can't live without one.

Accessible PDAs come in different formats: braille output, text-to-speech output, or a combination of the two. Your choice depends on whether you want to get your information in a tactile or audio format, or both. The bonus of a braille-based notetaker is that it has a built-in refreshable braille display, which lets you read and write braille. Of course, if you don't know braille, opt for the audio version with a QWERTY keyboard.

Notetakers also connect to your computer and can be used in place of your braille display or QWERTY keyboard. You must be using a screen reader for a notetaker to work effectively with your computer. Once the device is connected, files or information from the Internet, as well as information stored on the computer, can

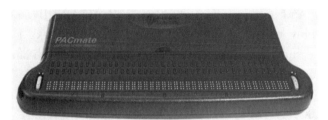

PAC Mate PDA With Forty-cell Braille Display. Notetakers such as Freedom Scientific's PAC Mate are multitasking devices that can do everything a regular PDA does. (Source: Photo courtesy of Freedom Scientific.)

be directly transferred onto the device for reading via the braille display or text-to-speech output.

Accessible PDAs and notetakers include Freedom Scientific's PAC Mate, HumanWare's BrailleNote and VoiceNote, and GW Micro's Braille Sense and Voice Sense.

TIP *If you don't have an accessible PDA, an accessible laptop will function just as well. An accessible laptop might be a good choice for someone with low vision who also wants a monitor to support visual display.*

Accessible Cell Phones

Accessible cell phones allow full access to nearly all of the phone's functions, including text messaging, e-mail, and Web browsing, through a screen reader.

In June 2009, Apple announced that it had added VoiceOver, its proprietary screen reader, to the iPhone—the first smartphone to have a built-in screen reader that is controlled by touching the screen. HumanWare and Code Factory also just released Orator, a screen reader for the BlackBerry.

In addition, many phones that operate on the Windows Mobile and Symbian platforms are compatible with third-party screen readers and screen magnifiers. For example, Code Factory makes screen-reader software called Mobile Speak. If you're an AT&T customer, AT&T will provide Mobile Speak on an AT&T phone for $89 as of this book's publication date. Meanwhile, Nuance makes

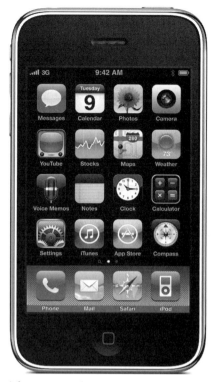

iPhone 3GS. Apple's iPhone 3GS is the first smartphone to have a built-in screen reader. It also has voice control. (Source: Photo courtesy of Apple.)

Nuance ZOOMS software that runs on Symbian-based phones, such as Nokia's, using its RealSpeak software speech synthesizers.

Alternatively, dozens of standard cell phones offer voice control for functions such as caller ID and status information. Though speech output is limited on these phones, many people who are blind are satisfied with these types of cell phones. Models include the LG VX5300, the Motorola i355, and the Samsung SGH-D357.

Braillers

Chances are that if you read braille, there will be a time when you want to create a hard-copy document in this format. Simple braille-writing devices such as the slate and stylus—akin to the pen and paper for sighted people—can be quite cumbersome. An alternative is a braillewriter, or brailler.

Like typewriters, braillewriters can be manual or electronic. An electronic braillewriter is more expensive but can include important functions such as text-to-speech. It's also easier to edit text and correct mistakes, and the device can be connected to a printer. Also helpful is the ability to connect the braillewriter to a QWERTY keyboard so that someone who cannot read braille can create a document for translation into braille.

In 2008, the Perkins School for the Blind and the American Printing House for the Blind announced the new Next Generation Perkins Brailler. The new version is lighter and less noisy than its predecessor and comes in eye-popping colors. The original Perkins Brailler was produced in 1951 at the Perkins School for the Blind.

TIP *Professionals who need to emboss their business cards can buy the Impressor, a custom-made embosser from the American Printing House for the Blind that will emboss up to four lines of braille on the back of a card. Regular business cards can also be shipped to Access-USA or another company to be embossed, for a fee.*

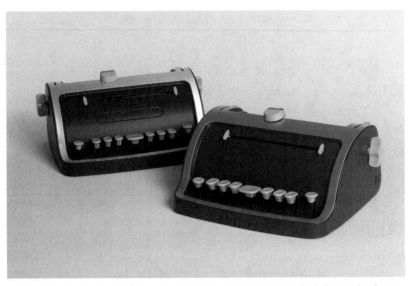

Next Generation Perkins Brailler. The Next Generation Perkins Brailler helps people who are blind to create physical documents in braille. (Source: Photo courtesy of Perkins School for the Blind and the American Printing House for the Blind.)

Scan/Read Software

Earlier in this chapter I mentioned how specialized scanning systems, which combine magnified text and OCR speech-to-text software, can be used by people who are visually impaired to enhance their reading skills.

A scanning system—often known as scan/read software—also provides a good solution for those who are blind and cannot read regular printed text. An image such as a book is digitally scanned, and OCR software allows the text to be accessed 100 percent auditorily using natural-sounding text-to-speech.

One of the most widely used scan/read systems is Kurzweil 1000, which is manufactured by Kurzweil Educational Systems.

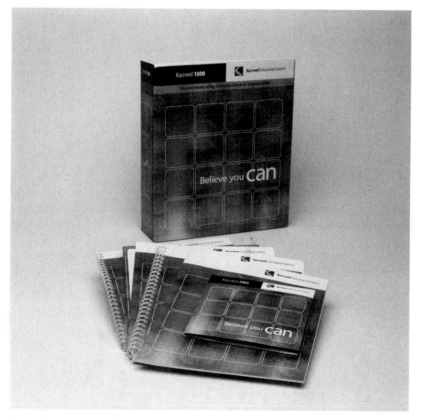

Kurzweil 1000. Kurzweil 1000 from Kurzweil Educational Systems is a scan/read program for those who cannot read printed text. (Source: Photo courtesy of Kurzweil Educational Systems.)

Kurzweil 1000 is an advanced reading software program. To use it, you'll need a computer system running Windows, a flat-bed scanner, a sound card, and the Kurzweil software. These components work together to produce natural-sounding speech in a variety of voices. Kurzweil 1000 also gives users the ability to write and edit documents, take notes, and complete simple forms independently. It can even burn CDs. Another great program is Freedom Scientific's OpenBook.

In 2008, knfb Reading Technology, a joint venture of Kurzweil Technologies and the National Federation of the Blind, debuted the smallest text-to-speech reading device to date for people with vision impairments. The knfbReader Mobile is a portable reading machine that works on a Nokia N82 cell phone with a

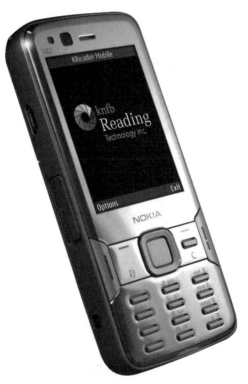

knfbReader Mobile. *The knfbReader Mobile from knfb Reading Technology is a portable reading machine that works on a Nokia N82 cell phone. (Source: Photo courtesy of knfb Reading Technology, Inc.)*

five-megapixel camera loaded with character-recognition and text-to-speech software.

The knfbReader Mobile can snap pictures of any printed material and read it aloud on the spot, including a book, e-mail, restaurant menu, receipt, or sign. It can even read U.S. currency to help blind people know whether they're using a $5 or $20 bill.

The Nokia N82 is also an accessible phone when used with a screen reader, so users can make and receive calls, access their contacts and calendars, and use the global positioning system (GPS).

The Great Inventor

Ray Kurzweil is a thirty-year pioneer in the field of assistive technology who developed the first-ever print-to-speech reading machine for the blind in the 1970s. The first Kurzweil Reading Machine covered an entire tabletop. On the day of the machine's unveiling, January 13, 1976, *CBS Evening News* anchor Walter Cronkite used the machine to give his signature sound-off, "And that's the way it was, January 13, 1976." While listening to NBC's *The Today Show*, musician Stevie Wonder heard a demonstration of the device and purchased the first production version, beginning a lifelong friendship between Wonder and Kurzweil.

Reading Machines

Standalone reading machines that scan and speak text without the use of a computer are still manufactured today by several companies. They are expensive, costing upwards of $2,500, and don't have the added features of a specialized scanning system.

Alternative-Format Books and Magazines

Every morning, Joe, who is totally blind, goes to Bookshare. org and downloads his daily newspaper, the New York Times. *He reads it in DAISY format on an accessible digital audio player, which provides both text-to-speech access for electronic files such as the newspaper or books and mp3 playback capability for music or audio files.*

DAISY stands for Digital Accessible Information System. It's a talking book file format that has special coding to allow users who are blind to bookmark a chapter, heading, or page, making it a more effective format than traditional mp3 files. DAISY works with screen readers on a computer, specialized DAISY players, and Scan/read software.

One of the best places to download DAISY books, as well as books in braille format, is Bookshare.org. Bookshare is one of the most prolific and innovative initiatives I've come across in my many years of writing about assistive technology. It's a searchable online library that offers more than 60,000 digital books, textbooks, and periodicals. The company is the brainchild of Jim Fruchterman, an engineer turned entrepreneur turned social activist. He started Bookshare after realizing that people who are blind or have other print disabilities, such as dyslexia, can take advantage of a copyright law exemption that gives people with qualifying disabilities free access to alternative formats of books.

Yes, any book publisher and author in the world must give the visual and print disabled full access to their books. That doesn't mean they have to do the heavy lifting: converting the books. Each book is painstakingly converted by volunteers into audio or braille format to help form the Bookshare collection.

Bookshare is free for qualifying students. Nonstudents can become members for $75 for the first year and $50 each year after that. They also must submit a proof of disability filled out by a certified professional.

If you qualify, you can also get free books in audio or braille format from the National Library Services for the Blind and Physically Handicapped, a division of the Library of Congress. The National Library Services is currently in the process of transferring its library of 16,000 titles from analog to digital format, a process that it says it will have completed by 2010.

Recording for the Blind & Dyslexic (RFB&D) is an audio textbook library that offers more than 30,000 free audiobooks, including math and science texts and literary classics, for qualifying candidates.

Alternative-Format Book Players

Downloading the digital book is only part of the equation. Anyone who wants to read a digital book must also have a reading device.

People who are blind can purchase a digital talking book player, or DAISY player, which will read aloud a book in DAISY format. It will also read mp3 books, such as those downloaded from Audible.com or the iTunes library.

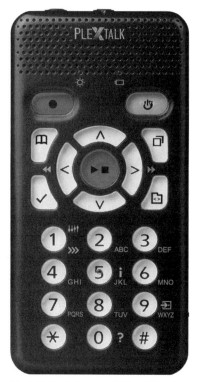

Plextalk Pocket. *Plextor's Plextalk Pocket is a DAISY-compliant music, voice, and book player and recorder. (Source: Photo courtesy of Plextor.)*

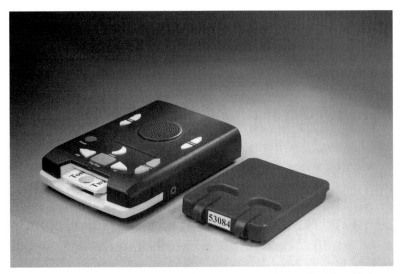

NLS Talking Book Player. *The National Library Services provides people with qualifying visual impairments with this free player to read audiobooks. (Source: Photo courtesy of the National Library Services for the Blind and Physically Handicapped.)*

HumanWare's Victor Reader Stream is the size of an iPhone and is packed with DAISY functions. Another company, Plextor, makes the Plextalk Pocket.

The National Library Services provides people with qualifying visual impairments with a free player to read audiobooks. The NLS digital talking books player has recently been updated; instead of using cassettes, it stores a single digital book on a flash memory card housed in a special cartridge. It will be available in the National Library Services' network of libraries starting in the summer of 2009.

Another option is to read DAISY books on your computer, laptop, or accessible PDA. For example, Freedom Scientific's PAC Mate notetaker can play DAISY books with special software, and in braille format using the refreshable braille display.

TIP *In 2008, Microsoft debuted a plug-in for its Word software program called "Save As DAISY.xml." This feature allows a Word user to save any document in the DAISY format to be read aloud on a computer or on a special DAISY player.*

Other Digital Book Libraries

A popular mainstream digital book library is Audible.com, where you can download books as mp3 files for a fee and listen to them on your mp3 player. There's also Apple's iTunes library, which has a good collection of mp3 audiobooks that can be downloaded for a fee. And Google has started to publish out-of-print works that can be downloaded online for free in mp3 format. Each of these sites is accessible via a screen reader.

Other Digital Book Players

The Kindle from Amazon is a popular mainstream digital book player that has received good reviews for its design and function but is inaccessible to people who cannot read text or see the menus and controls. Amazon attempted to add text-to-speech to its latest version to allow for "talking" books, but publishers expressed concern about copyright violations. As of today, some books downloaded on the Kindle, such as those from Random House, have had the text-to-speech function disabled by the publisher.

Travel Devices

For people who are blind, there are various devices that "talk" to provide information and directions. Among the newer technologies are GPS devices, which have already become popular among the driving public.

The GPS consists of twenty-four satellites orbiting the Earth. Commercial GPS devices are allowed to be accurate down to about thirty feet. GPS devices can help someone who is blind navigate streets to find locations and points of interest such as banks and restaurants. These devices are handheld and announce intersections as you walk. You can also record the names of landmarks.

For example, HumanWare makes the Trekker Breeze, which looks like a remote control. GPS is also available in some of HumanWare's other products, such as its accessible PDA, the BrailleNote.

Barcelona-based Code Factory makes Mobile Geo, a GPS solution for Windows Mobile smartphones and Pocket PCs. Mobile Geo can be integrated with Code Factory's screen reader, Mobile Speak.

Infrared systems are starting to surface as a way-finding technology. They use invisible infrared light, which is essentially an electromagnetic wavelength, to carry sound to receivers worn by listeners. This makes them a good solution for people who are blind and need assistance navigating unfamiliar public spaces such as airports. In fact, many U.S. airports are considering installing Talking Signs, an infrared system that communicates directional information to those carrying handheld receivers.

The Bank Note Reader from Brytech is a handheld device that can read aloud the denomination of U.S. banknotes. There's also a Canadian dollar version. Currencies in other countries, including the Japanese yen, the Swiss franc, and the Australian, Argentinean, Chinese, British, and Israeli currencies, have tactile systems for determining denominations.

Brytech also makes a color reader device that announces common colors plus tints and shades and that can tell whether your hotel room lights are on or off.

Household Devices

If you hoard canned goods, then you might like to use a home-made labeling system. At the very end of the spectrum are tactile pens with raised lines and dots, and braille label makers. However, there are a few higher-tech solutions.

You can use handheld barcode scanners in grocery stores and drugstores. A built-in database of more than 1 million products matches the barcode and speaks the name of the product. You can add information to the database. Freedom Scientific's ScanTalker costs $1,000 and works with its PAC Mate notetaker.

The i.d. mate II device from En-Vision America is an all-in-one handheld device that costs around $1,500 and doesn't require a computer or PDA to work.

There are also talking calculators, talking digital clocks and watches, and talking thermostats. Maxi-Aids and the Center for Independent Living both sell daily living aids.

Recreation

From braille bingo cards to tactile chess and checkers boards, there's no limit to the number of games that people who are blind can still enjoy. The American Foundation of the Blind's Web site (www.afb.org) has a full listing of games.

Some movie theaters offer audio descriptions of movies at certain times, and DVDs frequently include audio descriptions as well. These provide a helpful narrative that movie lovers can listen to along with the sound and script. You can check with movie theaters to find out what movies are playing with descriptive video service, or DVS.

Our vision can degenerate through the years. Someone who gets the most use out of low-vision products today may need more advanced, blindness-related technologies tomorrow.

Even sighted people can benefit from low-vision products if print and electronic information becomes too hard to read or comprehend as they age.

New technologies that are universally designed, such as accessible digital books players and cell phones, have the best potential for enhancing the lives of people with all ranges of vision.

Technologies for People with Hearing Disabilities

4

Deaf people can do anything a hearing person can, except hear.

—I. King Jordan

Of all the disabilities that I discuss in this book, deafness is the one with which I am most familiar. When I was four years old, I contracted spinal meningitis. As a result, I became profoundly deaf in both ears. I grew up wearing one hearing aid in my left ear but was totally deaf in my right ear.

In 2002 I received a cochlear implant made by a company called Advanced Bionics, one of three companies in the world that makes these devices. The cochlear implant provides an entirely different kind of hearing. It bypasses the damaged hearing nerves and sends sound waves directly to the brain.

Before we discuss devices that aid hearing, let's talk a little about hearing.

More than 30 million Americans are classified as hard of hearing. Not included in this group are older people who are starting to experience age-related hearing loss, which is also known as presbycusis. About 35 percent of people between the ages of sixty-five and seventy-five have some form of hearing loss.

Admitting to a hearing loss is often difficult. The situation is compounded by our sense of personal vanity: nobody wants to wear contraptions that scream "I can't hear!" Even in the early nineteenth century, manufacturers of hearing devices were making creative versions of early hearing aids, such as headphones and tubes worn underneath hats and wigs, chairs with built-in trumpets, and hearing devices for men that were disguised as water canteens.

Perhaps the most innovative hearing device is the one designed for King John VI of Portugal, who ruled in the 1820s. His throne was equipped with a large receiving apparatus concealed beneath the seat. The arms of the chair were hollow, and he forced people to kneel and speak into the chair so that he could hear them better. But he never told anyone he was hard of hearing!

In today's world, living with a hearing impairment isn't as hard as it used to be. Hearing aids have advanced from analog to digital devices, and they're small enough to wear behind the ear (BTE) or in the ear (ITE). (Remember the ubiquitous TV commercial for the miniature Miracle-Ear hearing aid?)

Communication with others is easier, too. Thanks to the Internet, we can use e-mail and instant messaging (IM) as our primary communication vehicles. We can also simply flip on the closed captions for a TV program or turn on subtitles for a DVD.

But that doesn't mean everything is easy. A hearing impairment can result in a lot of missed opportunities, from conversations to cultural events such as music concerts and movies. The good news is that a wide variety of assistive listening devices (ALDs) and assistive technologies exist to mitigate hearing loss for both aided and unaided users.

If you're experiencing hearing loss and not wearing a hearing aid, you might want to consider looking into one. Today's hearing aids are small and pack a powerful punch. Your doctor can refer you to an audiologist who can screen your hearing and recommend an aid that fits your individual needs.

If you're determined not to go the hearing aid route, there are a few solutions that will amplify sounds in cell phones, on television, and at the movies. Be sure to read the sections in this chapter on Technologies for Aid Users; you'll be happy to know that most of these products will also work for your needs.

Technologies for Non–Aid Users

Assistive listening devices include loud telephones, amplified handsets, headphones, headsets, and personal amplifiers. ALDs and other technologies help combat sound distortion, sound decay, and distracting background noise by transmitting undistorted sound directly to the listener. While there are a few multipurpose ALDs, the best ones target specific situations, such as listening to the TV, music from an mp3 player, computer audio, phone or cell phone conversations, meeting and lecture presentations, or stage shows and movies.

Loud Telephones

Katie is a thirty-one-year-old operations manager who has some hearing loss. When her boss gives an important presentation, Katie makes sure to bring along a Pocketalker Ultra personal listener. She places the microphone in front of her boss and wears earbuds so that his voice is amplified while background noises are reduced. For making telephone calls, Katie also uses an amplified telephone.

Non–aid users will want to get at least a telephone with amplification capabilities. Many of these phones amplify sound in the range of thirty to fifty decibels and provide noise-canceling features.

Clarity makes a large line of excellent amplified phones, some of which are available in RadioShack, Wal-Mart, and other stores. These phones range from the simple Clarity Amplified Trimline Phone to the Clarity Professional cordless amplified phone, which has dual speakers and a digital answering machine.

In addition to Clarity, VTech and Audex make several high-quality amplified cordless phones.

If you need a conference phone for work, a good choice is Polycom's SoundPoint Pro Full-Duplex Speakerphone, which combines a high-volume speakerphone with an amplified handset. Another business phone is the Fanstel Two-Line Amplified Speaker Business Phone with speaker. The phone's level of amplification has been tuned so that it more effectively restores the perception of many phonemic distinctions common in speech; your colleagues may not even be able to tell that you have a hearing loss.

Cell phone users should look to buy a model that has a loud receiver. Try them out at your wireless provider's stores. LG's VX models are known to have louder-than-average receivers. Clarity also makes the ClarityLife C900 Amplified Mobile Phone.

> **TIP** *Caller ID is one example of a mainstream technology that provides excellent benefits to the hearing impaired; the person receiving the call can decide whether they want to pick up the phone, and caller ID helps establish the context of the conversation before you answer the call.*

Amplified Handsets

Sometimes, using your own phone in the workplace isn't an option. Large corporations often have integrated communications networks that work only with certain telephones.

If you can't bring your own phone to work, you can try purchasing an inline telephone amplifier that attaches directly to a phone and will work with most telephones. Serene Innovations' business phone amplifier works with "virtually all business

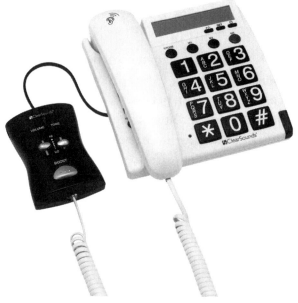

Portable Phone Amplifier. *The ClearSounds portable phone amplifier boosts the volume and clarity of the telephone. (Source: Photo courtesy of ClearSounds.)*

telephones" and boosts the volume up to 170 times. ClearSounds and Clarity make portable telephone amplifiers that are sold at Walgreens and Best Buy.

Generally, portable amplifiers don't work well on cell phones. If you have a cell phone, look into amplifiers that plug into the base of the phone and are used in conjunction with a headset. A good one to try: the Clarity Professional Mobile Headset Amplifier, which works with a Plantronics headset.

Alternatively, your company can probably order a custom volume-control handset from its telecommunications provider.

For outside of the office, you might want to use a portable, strap-on amplifier. This small battery-operated device isn't as powerful as an inline handset but is quite useful on a variety of cordless and regular phones and for traveling. Try the Megaphone Handset Amplifier from Global Assistive Devices.

Many of these accessories can be found on the Harris Communications Web site (www.harriscomm.com).

Headphones and Headsets

Headphones or a headset can do wonders in terms of reducing background noise in the office. People tend to listen to the phone with one ear, but for a person with some hearing loss, using two ears for phone conversations can offer a considerable benefit. Another big advantage over speakerphones and conference phones is the dimension of privacy.

Sony, Able Planet, Panasonic, and Bose make headphones with noise-canceling features. Plantronics is also a large maker of noise-canceling headsets. David Pogue, technology writer for the *New York Times*, thinks Panasonic's RP HC500 noise-canceling headset sounds just about as good as the twice-as-expensive Bose pair.

When shopping for an amplified home phone or office phone, choose one that has a headset socket and a headset selection button that allows the phone to be used without lifting the receiver. Office phones generally have proprietary headset sockets, which means they will accept only headsets that are compatible with those of the phone's manufacturer.

Personal Listeners

A newer technology available for non-aid users is the personal amplifier, also known as the personal listener. These devices are slightly larger than an mp3 player and are a good choice for amplifying sounds if you're not ready for a hearing aid.

Personal listeners use digital and analog technology and an external microphone to boost only the closest immediate sound source in the room. This helps bring out speech and music in difficult listening situations, while reducing background noises. Wearing earphones, you can also use the system for watching TV or listening to music; a separate jack lets you use it to amplify telephone calls.

When you use a personal listener, the most important factor to consider is how close the microphone can be placed to the sound source. The closer you can get, the greater will be the sound clarity and comprehension. Also, most personal amplifiers use an omnidirectional microphone, which picks up sound from all directions. These devices are more effective when they are used with a unidirectional microphone, which targets a specific area. For workplace meetings, the best solution is a boundary microphone, which picks up reflected sound from a conference room table.

The Pocketalker Ultra from Williams Sound offers the versatility to use a variety of directional, lapel, or boundary microphones to extend the device's use. The Bellman Audio Maxi has a built-in omnidirectional microphone. For more money—usually double what you'd pay for a wired solution—you can buy a wireless version, such as the Comlink Personal Sound Enhancer, which is worn on the ear.

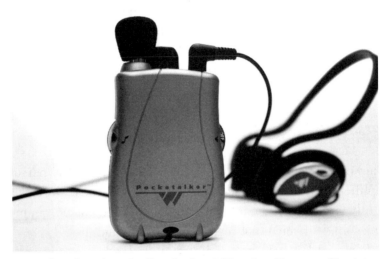

Pocketalker Ultra. *The Pocketalker Ultra from Williams Sound is a personal hearing amplifier that helps people with hearing loss communicate better. (Source: Photo courtesy of Williams Sound.)*

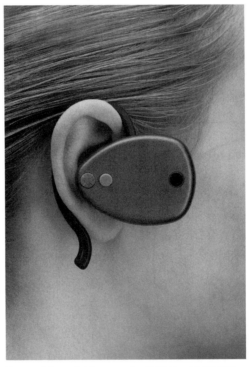

Personal Sound Enhancer. *Comlink's Personal Sound Enhancer is worn on the ear, in the same way as a headset. (Source: Photo courtesy of Comlink.)*

Technologies for Aided Users

Carol just turned sixty-five. She was fitted with a hearing aid after realizing she was missing a lot of what her husband was saying to her. She also had to turn up the volume very high on the television in order to hear it. An audiologist recommended a small, in-ear hearing aid for Carol that is nearly invisible. Her family and friends have noticed a remarkable difference in her ability to respond and understand. She wishes she had gotten a hearing aid sooner!

Hearing aids and, more recently, cochlear implants are two of the most powerful aids—or assistive technologies—for hard-of-hearing and deaf individuals.

True hearing aids have been around for more than 100 years. They are essentially sophisticated microphones that amplify sound. Today's devices use more advanced digital technology to boost sound and reduce background noise. A hearing aid is designed for a range of hearing loss from mild to severe to profound. A simple, in-the-ear (ITE) hearing aid can help someone who is older and is just starting to experience a slight loss of sound, while a more powerful, behind-the-ear (BTE) hearing aid can significantly boost hearing for those with severe to profound hearing loss and make the difference as to whether they are able actively to participate in society.

Cochlear implant processors, known as CIs, are a much newer technology. They are surgically implanted electronic devices that provide a sense of sound to a person who is profoundly deaf or severely hard of hearing. In addition to the internal device, which is implanted beneath the skin of the skull, there's an external headpiece that includes a microphone and speech processor. The internal and external components connect via a round magnet behind the ear.

Unlike hearing aids, cochlear implants do not amplify sound but work by directly stimulating any functioning auditory nerves inside the cochlea with an electric field.

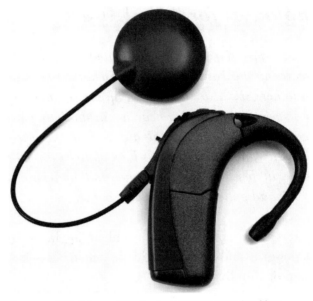

Harmony BTE. *Advanced Bionics manufactures several cochlear implant processors, including the behind-the-ear Harmony. (Source: Photo courtesy of Advanced Bionics.)*

About 400,000 people in the United States are considered deaf, meaning they have a profound or total hearing impairment. A large percentage of this group use assistive technology to hear. Approximately 150,000 people worldwide have received cochlear implants, with recipients split almost evenly between children and adults. Because of the high cost of the device, surgery, and post-implant therapy, the vast majority of users are in developed countries, although many health insurance programs cover the costs.

Sometimes, not even the use of a hearing aid or cochlear implant is enough for us to pick up all the sounds that we need to respond to throughout the day. For example, hearing aids pick up a lot of background noise, making "perfect" hearing impossible. These devices also must be removed at bedtime, so people who are deaf will not be able to hear an alarm clock or smoke detector. Hearing aids and cochlear implants can't get wet, either—so don't try to swim with one!

For these reasons, people who use hearing aids or cochlear implants can also benefit enormously from additional assistive technologies that enhance the capabilities of these devices when extra assistance is required.

ALDs interface with hearing aids—and, in some cases, cochlear implants—via FM radio, telecoils, direct audio input, or newer, proprietary communications gateways designed to interface with specific brands of hearing aids.

Telecoil

Of all these interfaces, the most important one for everyday use is the telecoil. The telecoil, or t-coil, is a small coil of wire that serves as an antenna and is built into many hearing aids and cochlear implants. The t-coil works with a variety of appliances, from cell phones, radios, and televisions to mp3 players and assistive listening systems.

When manually set to the t-coil position, a hearing aid's or cochlear implant's ambient microphone is disabled, which gives the advantage of blocking out 100 percent of the background noise. CIs and newer hearing aids may offer a program called M+T, which stands for microphone and telecoil. This program uses the t-coil while still making you aware of certain environmental sounds. For example, you can talk on the telephone using the t-coil and you'll still hear the doorbell ring.

Telephones and Cell Phones

Nick grew up with a hearing aid for most of his life. When he turned eighteen he made a decision to get a cochlear implant in one ear. Nick was amazed at the difference in clarity and sound. He loved that his audiologist could input unique programs into his device to provide more frequencies and balance sound levels. Today Nick is able to use a cochlear implant–compatible cell phone and a NoiZfree headphone adapter to listen to his iPod. He would never have been able to hear these devices with just his hearing aid.

Hearing aid or cochlear implant users must consider the compatibility of phones and cell phones, which should meet certain technical parameters to ensure the phone will work with their aid.

Phones may be called hearing aid or cochlear implant compatible; cell phones will have an M (microphone) or T (telecoil) compatibility rating. It's also desirable to choose a cell phone with an M3, M4, T3, or T4 rating from the Federal Communications Commission (FCC). Cell phones with lower ratings or no rating are unlikely to offer satisfactory compatibility with many hearing aids and may cause annoying interference.

Not all phones that are hearing aid or cochlear implant compatible work well with all hearing aids and cochlear implants. Trial and error—trying out phones at the store and asking about the store's returns policy—is the best way to ensure you'll be able to hear on a particular phone.

TIP

The Web site www.phonescoop.com has a list of hearing aid compatible phones from such manufacturers as Samsung, LG, Motorola, and RIM that you can access through its "Phone Finder" search.

Telephone Accessories

If you don't mind carrying around a few accessories, you can significantly enhance the volume and clarity on your phone or cell phone.

Ear Hooks and Neckloops

When used with a telecoil, ear hooks and neckloops help reduce noise interference and, in many cases, allow for hands-free use of your phones (and also work great for Skype calls). If you wear two hearing aids or two cochlear implants, then you'll want to get devices that work with both aids. Neckloops automatically work with two aids; ear hooks come in two models—single ear or dual ear—so get the dual-ear version if you wear two aids.

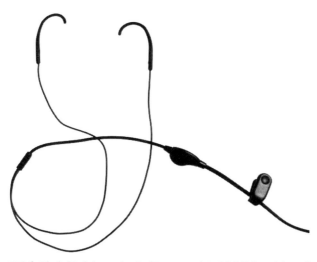

T-Link. *The behind-the-ear hook of Sensorcom's T-Link is lightweight and thin. It has a built-in microphone for hands-free calling. (Source: Photo courtesy of Sensorcom.)*

Ear hooks, also known as ear links, are worn behind the ear and tend to be more powerful than neckloops because of their close proximity to the telecoil. They are light and thin and don't take up much space behind the ear. British company Sensorcom's T-Link and T-Loop gadgets are well regarded. They are essentially hands-free cell phone kits that have a built-in microphone and look just like the hands-free kits used by hearing people.

A neckloop is worn loosely around the neck and has a cord that plugs into the device to which you are listening. Neckloops are easier to take on and off and can be hidden under your clothing. They are a better option if you don't like wires dangling down from your ears or if you wear eyeglasses and don't have any spare "ear real estate."

Since neckloops aren't as powerful as ear hooks, they are a better option for moderate hearing loss. Or you may want to consider an amplified neckloop to give you an extra boost of sound for telephone calls, such as ClearSounds' Amplified Power Neckloop.

You can also use a t-coil ear hook or neckloop to make Internet phone calls. NoiZfree PC plugs into your computer's soundcard

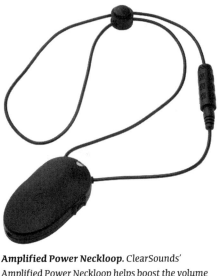

Amplified Power Neckloop. *ClearSounds' Amplified Power Neckloop helps boost the volume on telephone calls. (Source: Photo courtesy of ClearSounds.)*

sockets. You can then use it for voice over Internet protocol (VoIP) phone calls via Skype or MSN Messenger.

Bluetooth

By now you've probably heard of Bluetooth. Simply put, Bluetooth is short-range wireless technology, similar to your TV's remote control. Bluetooth provides a universal way to connect and exchange information between devices such as cell phones and headsets, and simplifies the discovery and setup of services between devices.

The advantage of using an ear hook or neckloop with a Bluetooth transmitter/receiver is that you'll have easy wireless and hands-free use of your Bluetooth-enabled phone or computer. For example, you can use a Bluetooth neckloop to clearly hear an incoming call directly through your aid and speak hands-free to the caller. You can also use Bluetooth to listen wirelessly to online radio stations from your computer.

A few Bluetooth transmitters to consider are Artone's Bluetooth LoopSet, ClearSounds' Bluetooth Amplified Neckloop, and NoiZfree's Beetle H-2ST Stereo with neckloop and single or twin stereo ear hooks.

TIP

If you have a cochlear implant from Advanced Bionics you can purchase a T-Mic microphone auxiliary ear hook. (This is not to be confused with a t-coil.) The T-Mic is a small ear hook with a microphone at the end that attaches to your cochlear implant. The benefit of a T-Mic is that it allows you to use a standard Bluetooth earpiece and not one that's specifically for t-coil users, which would be more expensive. There are a few inexpensive standard headsets on the market from Motorola and Sony for around $40.

Music and Other Audio Accessories

Ear hooks and neckloops can also be used for listening to mp3 players, DVDs, or the television. Before you buy either, though, decide whether hearing true stereo sound is important to you.

Stereo allows you to hear different sounds—different musical instruments, say—in each ear. While the output of almost all ALDs is mono (left or right), the output of almost all mainstream audio devices—radios, computers, iPods, and the like—is stereo. If you have two hearing aids and listen to these mainstream devices, then you will likely want stereo capability.

With dual ear hooks, if you are plugged into a stereo audio system you will hear true stereo sound, or separate channels for each ear. If you have hearing in only one ear, you can get a single ear hook that "merges" the two channels together so that nothing is lost. Good options are NoiZfree's iNoiZ-Music and Sensorcom's Music-Link. These devices can be purchased online at TecEar (www.tecear.com). If you prefer neckloops, try the NoiZfree NeckLOOP or Geemarc's iLOOP Powered Neck Loop; both deliver stereo left and right channels, so you hear the complete recording.

Assistive Listening Systems

Assistive listening systems (ALSs) are systems that interface with a telecoil and either a neckloop or ear hook and are used primarily between two or more people. ALSs include FM, loop, and infra-red systems, among others. These systems are quite powerful and work incredibly well in public places such as churches, court-rooms, movie theaters, and classrooms.

FM Systems

While I was growing up, I used an FM system in school. I still remember my first grade teacher, Mrs. Neefus, pulling me aside to give me a present that she had sewn herself. It was a colorful, strawberry-patch-patterned pouch for holding my FM system. I proudly wore it to school every day.

An FM system is a wireless communications system that helps a hearing-impaired person in difficult listening situations, such as a classroom. A radio microphone worn by the speaker (the teacher in this case) transmits radio signals to an FM receiver worn by the listener (the student) in the form of a neckloop or small "shoe" attached to the listener's hearing aid or cochlear implant.

Nobody else hears the amplified voice, just the FM user. This makes it a popular device in schools, places of worship (between pastor and churchgoer), and other one-on-one situations. At an office meeting, the radio microphone can be passed around to each speaker.

COMTEK, Phonic Ear, Williams Sound, Comfort Audio, and Phonak are all makers of FM systems for both personal listening and large-area situations. The Comfort Contego and COMTEK AT 216 are two self-contained systems worth looking into.

TIP *An FM system is a radio device that communicates on specific channels. If you are traveling internationally, you may have compatibility issues unless you are taking a self-contained system with you. Ask your audiologist for a list of countries where an FM system is approved for use.*

Sound Field Systems

A sound field system is a lot like an FM system and is generally used in classrooms where there is more than one child who is hard of hearing. They are basically Public Address systems with the inclusion of a wireless microphone. The teacher talks into the microphone or the microphone can be set up in the middle of a small group. The sound is sent to specialized receivers placed around the room that provide an extra eight or ten decibels of amplification. The system benefits children with hearing loss as well as children who hear normally.

Loop Systems

Audio frequency induction loop systems, known simply as loop systems, are a terrific technology. In public places where sound is broadcast over a microphone or speaker system, the loop system takes the sound straight from the source and delivers it right to a hearing aid or cochlear implant via a t-coil. The sound is also automatically adjusted to the frequency levels in your hearing aid or cochlear implant.

European countries are much more advanced than the United States in providing loop systems to their citizens; in London, for example, all the taxis and Underground ticket windows are looped for use with t-coil. Why has the United States lagged behind Europe? National healthcare systems in many European countries provide free or low-cost hearing aids to their citizens as part of health services. American insurance companies generally don't cover hearing aids, and it's estimated that only around 45 percent of Americans who wear hearing aids have a telecoil, though this is changing.

If you don't wear a hearing aid or you don't have the t-coil switch, you can still use a loop system via a portable receiver and headphones. Most people are unaware of their availability, unwilling to fuss with a new device, or averse to being seen as hearing impaired.

The guidelines in the Americans with Disabilities Act (ADA) for buildings and facilities require that buildings with fixed seating for fifty or more people have a permanently installed assistive listening system. A loop system is a cost-efficient way of meeting this requirement. Theaters, auditoriums, churches, lecture halls, and movie theaters all can be wired with a cable, resulting in a lower cost per user over time. People with hearing aids or cochlear implants just need their t-coil switch; those who don't have telecoil-equipped aids can use a portable receiving unit and a headset.

A loop system can also be installed in your home or a small conference room. Setup is easy. A chair pad loop kit, such as the Univox DLS-50 induction loop amplifier, is a thin pad that slips under a cushion and can cost as little as $200. The chair can be up to 30 feet from the amplifier, making it makes a great, semi-portable listening system for TVs, stereos, and telephones because it can be moved around a room.

You also have the option of looping your entire room with wire if you would like to enjoy your TV from any location within a looped area.

Infrared Systems

An infrared, or IR, system is an alternative to the FM system. It uses invisible infrared light waves to transmit sound to receivers worn by listeners. The advantage is that infrared requires line of sight, which makes it well suited to courtrooms and multiplex cinemas, where signals must be secure and not spill over into another room.

With infrared, the hearing aid or cochlear implant user wears a receiver and hears only the sound that comes from the infrared system. The device can also be worn as a set of headphones without a hearing aid.

Even with the options provided by assistive listening systems, many people with hearing aids and cochlear implants still rely on their good old telecoil transmitter. "Telecoil has some limitations, but it's cheap, highly beneficial, and a universal standard. It works the same anywhere in the world. Contrast that to FM or IR, where transmission frequencies vary from one system to another and are completely different in other countries due to lack of international agreements on standardization," says Paul Willington, president of TecEar, a hearing technology consultancy based in Southfield, Michigan.

Communications Gateway Devices

Hearing aid manufacturers are moving toward products that integrate more easily with a hearing aid. An ideal integrated system is one where, for example, a phone call would be prioritized over TV audio until the call had ended, and then the audio would

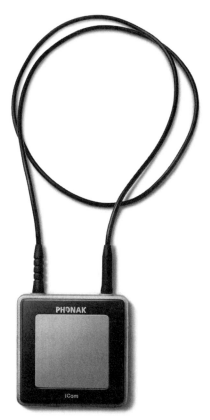

iCom. Phonak's iCom integrates your Phonak hearing system with virtually any audio source. (Source: Photo courtesy of Phonak.)

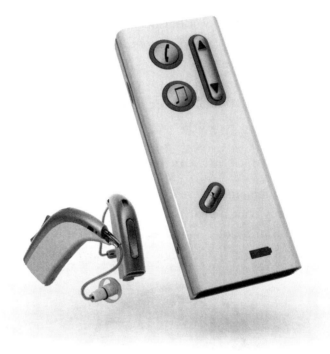

Epoq Streamer. *Oticon's Streamer is a compact Bluetooth device that acts as a gateway between Oticon's hearing aids and external sound sources. (Source: Photo courtesy of Oticon.)*

automatically be returned to the TV. Mainstream Bluetooth headsets for music cell phones already can perform this prioritization.

Hearing aid manufacturers have been moving toward integration via their proprietary wireless communications gateways. Essentially, these are Bluetooth devices that act as a gateway to provide direct audio connectivity between a hearing aid and audio sources such as music players, phones, and televisions.

For example, the Oticon Streamer works with Oticon's hearing aids. This fashionable gadget looks like an iPod (without the screen); it is carried in your pocket or worn around your neck and can activate up to eight Bluetooth devices. Phonak makes a similar transmitter, called the iCom, that is compatible with several of its hearing aids. Siemens makes the Tek for use with its own hearing instruments. These systems cost around $4,000.

While proprietary communications gateways offer greater integration, they are tied to one particular product: the user's hearing aid. Also, communications gateway devices won't provide access to loop systems, such as those used at meetings and conferences.

Alerting Devices

Assistive alerting devices are a nonaudio alternative to mainstream alarm systems that alert a person who is deaf or hard or hearing to an important sound, such as an alarm clock, doorbell, telephone, smoke detector, carbon monoxide detector, or baby's cry. As such, these devices can be lifesavers in many instances.

Alerting devices generally work with light or vibrations, often connecting a receiver to a lamp and wirelessly alerting you to sounds by flashing the lamp on and off. You can also buy receivers with built-in strobe lights that plug into wall outlets for rooms without lamps, such as the bathroom or garage.

Alternatively, you can wear a personal alert receiver, which has added benefits. It gives you more freedom to walk around the home and can vibrate in your pocket to alert you to a sound. You can also take a personal receiver with you when you travel.

Doorbell Signalers

There are many doorbells on the market that are designed for the deaf and hard of hearing. In some cases, a wireless doorbell is installed outside the door, and the receiver (chime), which is plugged into an electrical outlet located inside the home, flashes when someone presses the bell. Some units can be made to operate with the type of intercom system often found in apartments. When the intercom buzzer is pushed at the main door of an apartment building, the sensor inside the apartment will "hear" the sound and send a signal to a receiver.

Another type of device is attached to the inside of the door and responds to someone knocking by flashing a light. This type of device is best used in a small apartment or hotel room.

Alarm Clock Signalers

Alarm clocks are part of life; many of us can't wake up without them. There are both electrical alarm clocks and battery-powered alarm clocks, which are good for traveling. If you're hearing impaired, you can wake up to any combination of loud pulsating audio alarm, flashing lights, and shaking bed (in the latter case, a small vibrating device is placed under the pillow or mattress).

Sonic Alert makes the Sonic Boom, a combination flashing-vibrating alarm clock that is "guaranteed to wake even the heaviest sleepers." It gives you three different options for waking up: by lamplight, vibrator, or an adjustable buzzer. Clarity makes a similar device called the Clarity Lamp Flasher–Bed Shaker Combo.

Some devices have built-in AM/FM radios or the ability to flash a strobe light instead of connecting to a lamp. Small timers are also available, as well as wrist watches that use vibration as an alarm or alert.

Smoke and Carbon Monoxide Detectors

There are two options for smoke and carbon monoxide safety. The first is to make existing conventional smoke and carbon monoxide detectors accessible by mounting a sound-monitoring device close to the detector. When the detector alarm goes off, the sound monitor "hears" the sound and sends a signal to a receiver in order to activate a bed shaker or flash a strobe light or lamp.

The second option is to use a special smoke and carbon monoxide detector that sends a signal to a bed shaker or flashes a strobe light or lamp.

The ADA requires that all workplaces provide visual equivalents to their smoke detector systems.

Baby Monitors

If you have small children, you probably need to have a baby monitor. Hearing-impaired parents can use baby monitors that alert them to a baby's cry in a variety of ways.

Many parents who are deaf or hard of hearing choose video monitors, also known as baby cams. The receiver can be plugged into a TV or can include a portable LCD screen. Some baby cams can work at night with low light levels or have a night-vision feature.

Graco's imonitor Video Vibrating Baby Monitor has a range of up to 600 feet. Alternatively, the imonitor (without video) is a wearable baby monitor that vibrates or flashes. It has a range of up to 2000 feet.

If you have more than one child and need to monitor two rooms, the Summer Infant Two-Room Scanning Video Baby Monitor is worth a look.

The AlertMaster AMBX Baby Monitor by Clarity is a wireless transmitter that you place in your bedroom. It can connect to a lamp or vibrating alarm clock—the receiver—to alert you to the sound of your child's cries.

Another monitoring system, the Why Cry Baby Crying Analyzer, is unique because it can recognize the variations among types of cries and identify them for you. Common cries are analyzed and summarized in five mood categories: hungry, bored, annoyed, sleepy, and stressed.

Telephone Signalers

A phone with an amplified ring volume or tone may be all you need for your hearing aid. You might also benefit from a flashing light on your phone. Some people like to use a combination amplified ringer and strobe light that flashes on an incoming call.

Serene Innovations' Super Loud Phone Ringer/Flasher has audible and visual alerts that are activated when there is an incoming phone call. You can plug in an optional bed shaker for nighttime alerts.

Omni-Page makes a telephone kit that uses vibration. The kit plugs into a phone jack, and you wear a small device that vibrates on an incoming call.

Many multiuse alerting systems include telephone signalers.

Multiuse Alerting Systems

A popular option among the hard of hearing is to purchase a multiuse alerting system. You typically buy a base unit, or receiver, and purchase the signalers you need for your home separately.

The Alertmaster AM-6000 Notification System by Clarity provides alerts to telephone calls and the doorbell. This system can be expanded by adding optional accessories such as a baby cry monitor and a motion detector. It comes with a bed shaker and a wireless doorbell transmitter.

Sonic Alert, a large provider of signaling devices, makes a multiuse system that includes a wireless three-room signaling system for the doorbell, phone, and alarm clock that plugs into a lamp. The system includes a Sonic Boom alarm clock with bed vibrator.

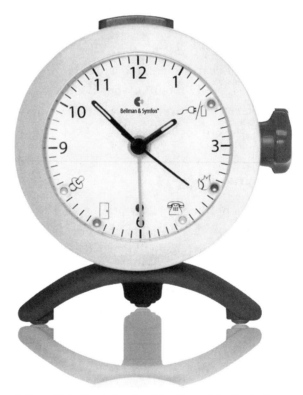

Bellman Visit. *The sleek and stylish Bellman Visit offers both visual and vibrating signals. (Source: Photo Courtesy of Bellman & Symfon Europe AB.)*

Design nuts will like the Swedish-designed Bellman Visit wireless alerting system, a multiuse system that lets you choose either a visual or vibrating signaler. The vibrating signaler is held in the pocket, while the visual signaler stands on a table. It also comes in the form of a wristwatch for an even more sophisticated waking experience.

Travel

There are many portable multiuse alerting systems that you can take along when you travel, but they are expensive and cost upward of $500. The Americans with Disabilities Act requires all U.S.

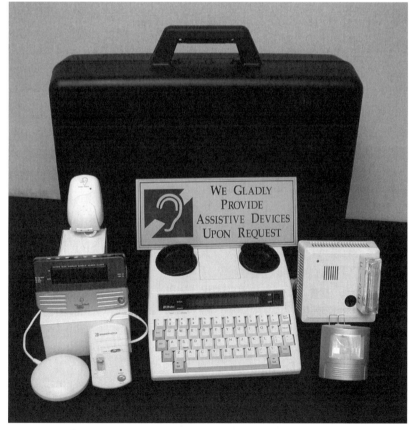

ADA 500 Hotel Kit. An ADA-compliant hotel kit includes a text telephone, wakeup system, and telephone signaler, among other devices. (Source: Photo courtesy of Harris Communications.)

hotels and motels (and even hospitals) to provide ADA-compliant devices for the deaf and hearing impaired free of charge to guests (and patients) who request them.

Hotels must provide a system that includes a text telephone, telephone signaler, telephone amplifier, door knock signaler, wakeup system, and visual/audio smoke detector. Some kits include a television decoder for closed captions, but today most televisions have built-in closed-captioning systems and these decoders aren't necessary. Hotel personnel can set up these systems for you ahead of your arrival, so be sure to ask for this kit at the time of booking. If you're traveling outside of the United States you may have to take your own kit and electrical current adapters.

Nonaudio Technologies for Aided Users

People with hearing impairments can make use of enhanced audio because they either have some natural hearing or use hearing aids and cochlear implants that amplify sound. But there are other ways to take in information that don't rely on audio alone. People who are totally deaf and do not wear hearing instruments can take advantage of many nonaudio technologies.

First, a little about deaf culture. Deafness is one of the few disabilities with its own culture. "Deaf culture" generally refers to the use of deaf people's native language, American Sign Language (ASL), as part of the advancement of deaf causes.

Sign language is a complete, complex, and visual language that uses signs made with the hands and other movements, such as facial expressions. American Sign Language is used by many deaf North Americans; other countries have developed their own languages that differ notably from ASL.

Even though ASL is used in America, it is a language completely separate from English. ASL has its own rules for grammar, punctuation, and sentence order.

A recent trend is to teach hearing infants a simple form of ASL called "baby sign," which is said to help parents converse with their children and socialize them into the world.

In the past thirty years, technological advances have ignited controversy within the deaf and hearing community over whether deafness is something that needs to be corrected—with a hearing aid or cochlear implant, for example.

In *Sound and Fury*, a PBS documentary that was nominated for an Academy Award for Best Documentary Feature in 2001, evidence of a strong deaf culture appears. The film documents one family's struggle over whether to provide their two deaf children with cochlear implants. The parents, who also were deaf, believed that deaf culture was under attack by advances made in bionic devices such as cochlear implants.

However, not everyone who is classified as deaf is part of deaf culture. It's very much a personal choice and a reflection of deaf language, community, and ideals.

In fact, some deaf people do not use sign language at all; they prefer to lip-read and speak orally. This is helpful for communicating with hearing people. Another option for deaf-to-hearing communication is the use of sign-language interpreters. Generally, these are professionals certified in American Sign Language who can translate conversations in real time. Interpreters might be on hand to translate a lecture, meeting, or doctor's appointment. They charge $100 to $200 an hour, often with a two-hour minimum, which makes this an expensive option.

Fortunately, there are a few workarounds to hiring a live interpreter if one isn't available. These solutions should by no means replace an interpreter, but they serve as reliable and inexpensive options for meeting the face-to-face needs of deaf people in certain situations.

iCommunicator is a software program that runs on a Windows computer. It uses a speech-to-text technology to translate conversations between deaf and hearing people, as well as between deaf people and people with vision loss (who may not be able to see sign-language signals). iCommunicator can translate speech to text, speech or text to video sign language, and speech or text to a computer-generated voice.

The best part is that there's no interpreter involved. The program has a database of sign language videos that includes 30,000 signed words and 9,000 video clips that can be strung together to create sentences—and conversations—from speech or text. The program uses Dragon NaturallySpeaking, an advanced text-to-speech engine.

How iCommunicator Works

Say a person who is deaf and uses sign language goes to his doctor's office for a checkup. He can use iCommunicator to sign what's been ailing him, and the computer will "speak" the results. The doctor nods and asks the patient some questions. The doctor, who has trained the computer to recognize her voice, wears a headset with a microphone to talk to the patient. iCommunicator translates those questions into video sign language on the computer screen. If a sign is unavailable, the word is finger-spelled.

Similar scenarios can be played out with colleagues and customers who are deaf.

iCommunicator costs $6,500 and, at the time of publication, is available on the Windows platform only.

Closed-Captioning

Closed-captioned television programs offer a way for deaf and hard-of-hearing individuals to "read" the dialogue and sound effects on a program. Closed-captioned programming is a relatively new technology. It started in 1980 with *Masterpiece Theater* and a few other programs, but it required a special television with a built-in closed-captioning decoder.

In the 1990s, the Federal Communications Commission adopted rules that required more and more programs to be captioned. Today, 100 percent of all new English programming (with certain exemptions for programming aired in early morning hours, among a few other minor exceptions) have captions, and by 2010 all Spanish language program providers will be required to provide Spanish captions, with minor exemptions. Captions can be turned on or off using the remote control or by going to your TV's settings menu.

Going to the movies has always been difficult for hard-of-hearing and deaf people. Movie theaters don't do a very good job of making sure the movies that they play are accessible to people with disabilities such as sight and hearing loss.

While assistive listening devices are available, people who lip-read or can't rely on audio alone would like to see captioned movies. In today's digital age, captions can easily be embedded in digital films as subtitles. However, movie chains don't turn them on, saying that they would inconvenience their nondisabled viewers.

Sometimes, movie theaters purchase open-captioned films and screen them at certain times of the day (usually during off-hours). Open captions are different from closed captions because open captions are a permanent part of the film and can't be turned off. For this reason, movie theaters generally don't purchase open-captioned films for the general public.

One solution that has been in operation for close to ten years throughout the United States is rear-window-captioning, a closed-captioning technology devised by the Media Access Group at WGBH in Boston. Rear-window-captioning involves an LED display in the back of the theater that projects dialogue onto a small plastic screen that sticks into the viewer's soda cup holder.

Read Any Good Movies, Lately?

"Two for Jurassic Park 3, please," I said to the ticket girl. It was a Tuesday night at the General Cinema Theater in Clifton, N.J., and I was about to "hear" my first blockbuster film. [In 2001] the theater [was] the only in the state to have installed the Rear Window Captioning System for the deaf and hard-of-hearing.

I've been profoundly deaf since the age of four and until now the only movies I could enjoy were those with subtitles—usually that meant the foreign ones. The ticket girl handed me my change, which didn't amount to much: As at Broadway plays and other artistic performances, deaf and hard-of-hearing persons rarely get a price break, even though they aren't absorbing the full experience. Alas, they really just buy seats to the show.

Jurassic Park wasn't my first choice, but captioning is set up for only one movie at a time, at the manager's discretion. So I picked up the Rear Window device at the customer-service desk. As my friend and I walked to our seats, all eyes were on us: This assistive technology wouldn't win any awards for its design. I felt like I had walked into a funeral parlor carrying a golf club.

Rear Window is a tinted square of Plexiglass attached to a bendable arm that is supposed to fit snugly inside your cup holder. (Where you're to put your soda, I'm not sure.) Mounted on the back wall is a digital panel that resembles an electronic stock-ticker board. When the film begins, the movie script is spelled out backwards on the back wall, and the Plexiglass—when adjusted oh-so perfectly—catches the words and reflects them for the reader.

It's not exactly quantum physics. My friend quipped that the technology is about one step removed from a guy holding up cue cards. It also took about 20 minutes of shifting and bending the arm to catch the captioning just right. But once there, voilà, I was set.

Being a wordsmith, my top concern with captions is the quality of writing. Hastily transcribed captions can sometimes strip away the flavor of language and expose a film's dependence on its script. Thriller dinosaur flicks like Jurassic Park are crafted with simple plots and lots of visual action, which gives the caption writers a chance to show off a little. In one scene, a battle royale between a T-rex and a spinosaur was described with lots of pizzazz: roar, snarly growl, neck ripping, bones crunching. No more T-rex.

In another scene, the paleontologists and their cohorts are locked inside an oversize birdcage with an angry flock of flying pteranodons, and there's all sorts of staccato growling, rhythmic cawing, loud hissing, crickets chirping, and other illustrations that drum up violent visions of winged carnivore vs. suburban soccer mom—sanitized, of course, for a PG-13 hearing-impaired audience.

Source: Reprinted from (August 22, 2001) issue of *BusinessWeek* by special permission, copyright © (2001) by The McGraw-Hill Companies, Inc.

Videotapes and DVDs do allow for closed-captioning, or they include subtitles, sometimes displayed in the settings menu as English, English Subtitles for the Deaf and Hard of Hearing, or English SDH. However, the newer HD-DVD and Blu-ray Disc media cannot have closed captions due to the design of the high-definition multimedia interface specifications. Thus, if the movie studio has included English or English SDH subtitles on the DVD, you won't have any problems, but if they have provided only closed captions, you won't be able to read them on an HD-DVD or Blu-ray Disc DVD player.

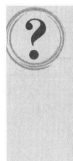 Today's TVs have closed-captioning decoders built into them, but that wasn't always the case. In 1990 the Federal Communications Commission passed the Television Decoder Circuitry Act, requiring all new televisions with screens of thirteen inches or larger to be able to receive and display closed captions. So when you go to the store to buy a new TV, your captioning needs are completely covered.

Computer-Assisted Note Taking

Meredith is a student in graduate school. She is hearing impaired and relies on notetakers to help her in classes. Meredith prefers real-time captioning because she doesn't like to miss anything that's going on in class, including students' questions, remarks, and jokes. Her husband, Jon, prefers more discrimination; he'd like his notetaker to focus only on the topic at hand rather than have to read through more pages of notes at the end of the day.

Computer-assisted note taking comes in many forms. Some programs are overarching, providing a verbatim transcript of everything that happens in a classroom or meeting, including other students' comments. Other programs are designed to take more focused notes on the core topic of a meeting or lecture. Generally, which program is used depends on what the student or employee prefers, as well as the associated costs of hiring a person to interpret the meeting or lecture.

Communication Access Real-Time Translation

Communication access real-time translation, or CART, is a service that has its origins in stenography; only it's a much more complex system. With CART, a verbatim transcript of a lecture or meeting is simultaneously created and transmitted by highly skilled CART provider using a stenotype system of shorthand notation. Special equipment immediately translates the codes into text, which is displayed in real time on a large screen or a computer monitor.

Captioning professionals can produce text at speeds of at least 225 words per minute, which is much faster than the speed of normal speech. CART can be used to transcribe court proceedings, conferences, lectures, weddings, and other events as they unfold. The text can also be saved and printed or published online.

CART requires both the computer hardware and a captioning professional who has trained for at least two years to learn how to operate the keyboard, making this an expensive option for schools and employers. It costs up to $200 an hour.

Chicago-area company Caption First provides CART services both locally and nationally through remote technology. You can also search the National Court Reporters Association's online CART Provider Directory at http://cart.ncraonline.org/Directory.

TypeWell and C-Print

TypeWell and C-Print are the names of two abbreviation typing software programs, which allow captionists to input text based on phonetics, which reduces keystrokes. C-print is a program developed at the National Technical Institute for the Deaf.

These note-taking systems are very similar in nature: notetakers use standard computer keyboards and word-processing software to create meaningful, spoken-English transcriptions of a lecture or meeting rather than a verbatim transcription. As a result, the notes are condensed and more concise. With C-Print Pro, a captionist can also provide C-Print speech-to-text services using a combination of the keyboard system and his or her voice.

TypeWell and C-Print have a top speed of about 120 words per minute with a very fast and accomplished operator, whereas CART providers have to be able to write at least 225 words per minute. However, both TypeWell and C-Print are less costly options because they're more widely available.

TypeWell and C-Print can be offered as remote services. Remote computer-assisted note taking (CAN) has gained popularity in recent years as high-speed Internet connections have become more ubiquitous. With remote CAN, the service provider is located elsewhere, often in another state, and is connected to the classroom or conference room by phone line or the Internet. A microphone in the room picks up the speaker's words, which are transmitted to the provider. The provider transcribes them, and the text is sent back for display on a computer at the person's desk or on a laptop. These systems have somewhat reduced reliability and can be quite a bit more expensive than local transcribing, but they're sometimes the best solution when the need for transcription comes up unexpectedly.

Voicewriting

Voicewriting is based on automatic speech recognition, and there are two types: professional and casual. Professional voicewriters are service providers who have taken courses in speech-to-text and may have been certified at a particular performance and accuracy level.

Casual voicewriting includes speech-to-text translation for a classroom teacher whose speech goes directly to the computer or by an employee who uses speech-recognition software, such as Dragon NaturallySpeaking, for a few weeks. An alternative that's used in a number of schools is Caption Mic by ULTECH. Caption Mic is a speech-recognition-based captioning system in which the user—a teacher, say—trains her own voice to use the program.

Caption Mic uses IBM's ViaVoice as its underlying engine and has a vocabulary of more than 200,000 words. The software can export a text document of the session and can also be used to caption online videos and DVDs.

If all else fails and no computer-assisted note-taking system is available, sign-language and oral interpreters can provide translations in a pinch—with no equipment necessary.

 Many museums around the country offer sign-language interpreters, CART, or similar services for their lectures. Be sure to call and request the service in advance.

Communications

Text Telephones

A text telephone (TTY) is a small typewriter that allows two individuals to communicate with each another over a standard telephone line by typing text back and forth. TTYs are available with memory and answering machine capabilities. They can store conversations as well as greeting messages. In addition, some TTYs have a built-in printer that can print a conversation as it proceeds.

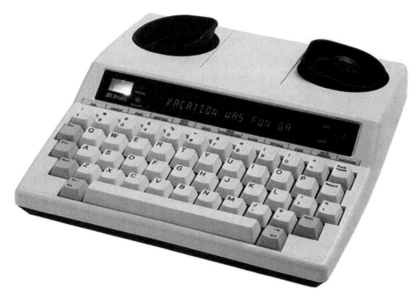

Text Telephone. Ultratech's Supercom 4400 is a text telephone that is specially outfitted for users who are deaf or hard of hearing. (Source: Photo courtesy of Ultratech.)

There are also portable TTYs available that can be used with cell phones. Public spaces such as government buildings, airports, and convention centers have TTYs on hand.

TIP

Most airports have TTY booths, but a few airports go above and beyond. Salt Lake City airport was the first to install videophone booths for deaf and hard-of-hearing travelers to make sign-language calls. Chicago's O'Hare and Midway airports have similar services. The nation's airports are also working toward installing gate monitors to show which rows are boarding, as well as interactive visual paging screens.

TTY Relay Service

When one party does not have a TTY, an operator can act as a typist during the conversation. The operator is employed by the FCC's Telecommunications Relay Service (TRS), which is available twenty-four hours a day, seven days a week, by calling 711 on your TTY machine.

For example, someone who is deaf and who uses a TTY can use the relay operator to call a hearing person. The relay operator acts as the bridge between the two parties, helping to relay both text and spoken words. People who use a TTY but prefer to use their voice instead of text can use a voice-carry-over TTY, where the relay operator listens to the deaf caller's voice but still types the hearing party's words.

Advances in instant messaging and Internet protocol technology have revolutionized communications for the deaf and hard of hearing: it's no longer necessary to make calls on a clunky TTY machine.

Internet protocol (IP) technology now lets deaf people make calls over their computer, cell phone, or PDA. For many years, the cell phone of choice for the deaf was the Sidekick from T-Mobile. It has a large screen and QWERTY keyboard, making it convenient for text messaging, instant messaging, and, of course, relay calls.

With today's cell phones becoming more sophisticated, deaf people now have more options. The iPhone, Google's G1, the BlackBerry Storm, and the Palm Treo Pre, among others, are vying for top place in the smartphone market. Each has its own version of a QWERTY keyboard and supports text messaging, IM, and relay calls.

In 2004 AOL and Hamilton Relay launched the AIM Relay Service free of charge to AIM users. The service can be accessed from any computer or wireless device running AIM (on a Windows computer) or iChat (on a Mac).

AIM now has partnerships with several relay service providers with unique AIM handles, including Purple Communications (i711relay and IPRelay handles), Sorenson IP Relay (SIPRelay handle), and Sprint Relay (Sprint IP handle).

Videophones

Another new technology is the videophone, which can be used for making sign-language calls. A few deaf-specific companies make videophones, including Purple Communications, Sorenson, and CSD. Videophones are getting smaller and smaller, and many have wireless capabilities for sending e-mails and browsing

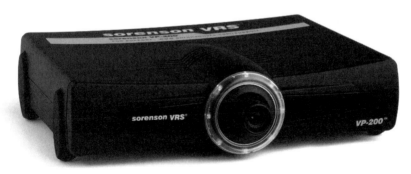

Photo provided courtesy Sorenson Communications.

VP-200 videophone. *The Sorenson VP-200 videophone is free for qualifying deaf and hard-of-hearing users for making sign-language calls. (Source: Photo courtesy of Sorenson Communications.)*

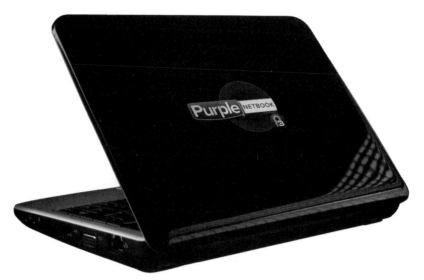

Purple Netbook. *Purple's Netbook is an all-in-one communications device for making video and text calls and performing other Web-based tasks. (Source: Photo courtesy of Purple Communications.)*

the Web. Videophones work with a high-speed Internet connection for video-to-video calling between two sign-language users.

In May 2009, Purple Communications introduced the Purple Netbook, a Windows XP laptop that has built-in videophone architecture, including a Webcam and Ethernet and Wi-Fi Internet access. Purple's P3 software includes Purple's video and text relay services, point-to-point video calling, and a shared address book. The software is free with the purchase of a Purple Netbook, a compact device that costs $200 after a discount for deaf and hearing-impaired customers.

Don't have a mobile videophone? Another good—and easy—option for mobile video calling is to use a laptop equipped with a Web camera and Internet connection. Again, two deaf people can connect directly and sign with one another using Skype or iChat.

If you're deaf or hard of hearing and use sign language, you can apply for a free videophone and video-conferencing software from many companies that provide video relay services. Try Sorenson, CSD, or Purple Communications, which operates the Hands On Video Relay Service.

Video Relay Services

With videophones, in order for a deaf person to talk to a hearing person (and vice versa), a relay service is required. In the United States, video relay services use a relay operator who is fluent in American Sign Language. VRS calls can take place through a videophone linked to a telephone line, on a mobile videophone, or over a computer using an audiovisual conference program such as AIM or iChat.

Three VRS companies that are well known within the deaf community are Sorenson, CSD, and Purple's Hands On Video Relay Service. Each company supplies videophone hardware and operates call centers staffed by sign-language interpreters. Salt Lake City–based Sorenson has a large share of the market, as it was the first to come out with videophones.

To make a call using the Sorenson VRS, a deaf caller uses a Sorenson videophone or a desktop or laptop with video-conferencing software (such as Sorenson EnVision SL or Microsoft NetMeeting) to dial the VRS call center. A sign-language relay operator pops up on the screen and places the call.

Likewise, a hearing person can place a video relay call to a deaf or hard-of-hearing person by dialing the videophone's unique phone number or calling the VRS call center.

While Sorenson doesn't support Macintosh computers, Hands On Video Relay Service provides VRS on the Mac using iChat.

> **?** The FCC has reserved the phone number 711 for access to TRS and VRS. The system is available 365 days a year, 24 hours a day, 7 days a week—and it is free. Spanish relay is also available: type "Hola" to let the relay service know you want to place a call in Spanish.

Video Remote Interpreting

Video remote interpreting, or VRI, uses a videophone or a computer with a Web camera to access sign-language interpreting services when there's no interpreter on site. VRI can be used in situations such as staff meetings, doctor visits, conferences, and training sessions.

Instead of an interpreter being physically present, the interpreter is located remotely and communicates live. This method saves companies such as banks, courtrooms, medical facilities, libraries, schools, and other businesses and organizations the cost of mileage, travel time, and two-hour minimums for in-person interpreting sessions. While the company still has to pay for interpreting services, it's a more cost-efficient option.

Captioned Telephones

A captioned telephone (CapTel) is conceptually similar to a captioned television. It's a custom telephone that allows people to receive word-for-word captions for their telephone conversations. A CapTel works like any other telephone but includes a display screen for the text.

When a caller used a CapTel, the call is connected—behind the scenes—to a relay service operator who provides the captioning. The CapTel service center's specially trained operator uses voice-recognition technology to transcribe whatever is said by the other party into text on the CapTel's five-inch color screen. The caller still hears the person's voice on the other end of the line. Spanish captions are also available.

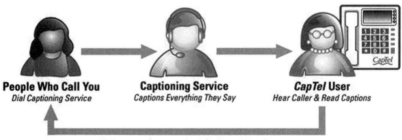

People Who Call You
Dial Captioning Service

Captioning Service
Captions Everything They Say

CapTel User
Hear Caller & Read Captions

Calls you make are automatically captioned.

How the CapTel Works. *A special telephone designed to work with a captioning service displays captions during your telephone calls. (Source: Photo courtesy of Ultratech.)*

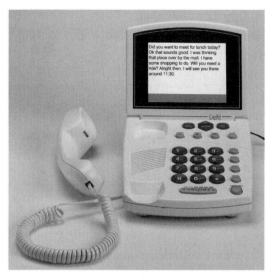

CapTel. With a CapTel phone, relay service operators use voice-recognition technology to transcribe calls. (Source: Photo courtesy of Ultratech.)

There's no cost for participating in the program, but you must buy a CapTel phone. The CapTel 200 works with traditional analog telephone lines. For the newest version of the CapTel, the CapTel 800i, you need a landline and a high-speed Internet connection.

Not all states have the CapTel program yet. However, an alternative version that's available nationwide is WebCapTel. This service is operated by both Sprint and Hamilton CapTel. It lets you use a standard telephone and view captions for the call in your computer browser. The captions are sent over the Internet.

E-mail and Visual Voicemail

While commercial e-mail has been around for more than two decades, it's one of the most transforming technologies for individuals who are deaf or hard of hearing. E-mail is a mainstream technology that doesn't reveal one's hearing loss, so it keeps a level playing field—which can be important in the business world.

E-mail is a great way to contact business associates and connect with family and friends, and it lets you keep a record of everything written.

A technology that has been slowly percolating through the workplace is visual voicemail. This adds an optical component to phone voicemail, such as allowing the user to view a list of voicemail entries and read transcriptions of voicemail. Several telecommunications companies have started integrating this service into their devices, including the iPhone and the BlackBerry Storm. In addition, technology vendors are planning to introduce visual voicemail programs, including Google Voice and RocketVox.

Technologies for the deaf and hard of hearing are a mix of old and new, and many live side by side. More versatile mainstream technologies, such as Web conferencing, are opening new listening and communications opportunities for people with hearing disabilities.

Many people who are deaf can remember a time when a TTY machine was the only way to connect with a hearing person. Recently, I watched an episode of MTV's *Truth* in which a deaf teenager lamented the fact that he was constantly having to text-message his friends. His thumbs were sore, perhaps? I wish texting had been available when I was young.

In the meantime, more assistive technologies, such as video relay and voice-recognition technology, are taking root. Soon the TTY machine might be collecting dust on the shelf to make way for a new age of innovation. All of these advances will continue to open up doors for people with hearing disabilities and enhance their work and life opportunities.

Technologies for People with Physical Disabilities

5

The fact is that even if your body doesn't work the way it used to, the heart and the mind and the spirit are not diminished.

—Christopher Reeve

Mike, an accountant, was diagnosed with multiple sclerosis when he was forty years old. At his offices, it's easier for Mike to use a scooter than to walk from meeting to meeting. Mike has trouble using his hands. Instead of typing on a keyboard he uses a speech-recognition program, and instead of holding a telephone he wears a headset.

Physical disabilities encompass a broad range of disabilities that affect a person's limbs, muscles, nerves, or motor skills. A physical disability may be congenital or acquired from disease or injury, or it may be brought on by a condition such as muscular dystrophy, multiple sclerosis, or cerebral palsy.

Physical disabilities also include conditions such as arthritis and fibromyalgia, which cause pain in the bones and can affect dexterity and motor skills. Other people may have hidden disabilities, such as a heart condition or epilepsy, that limit their ability to perform certain functions.

Someone with a physical disability may require one or more artificial limbs to get around. They may use a wheelchair, crutches, a cane, or a combination of these mobility aids. Or they may simply require alternative ways of performing daily tasks such as typing or talking on the telephone.

Paralysis is a common physical disability. Paralysis is the loss of the power to move some part of the body due to injury or disease. It's caused by damage to the brain or nervous system, and especially to the spinal cord.

President Franklin D. Roosevelt spent his entire presidency hiding the effects of childhood polio, which caused paralysis of his legs. Christopher Reeve, the actor who played Superman, was paralyzed by a spinal cord injury after being thrown from the horse he was riding in 1995. Until his death in 2004 at age fifty-two, Reeve was a staunch advocate for treatments and technologies for those living with paralysis, and his work continues through the Christopher and Dana Reeve Foundation.

More than 1 million Americans are paralyzed due to spinal cord injuries; about a half-million Americans live with multiple sclerosis, a chronic disease that attacks the central nervous system and can cause numbness in the limbs, paralysis, or loss of vision. Other causes of paralysis include stroke, trauma, cerebral palsy, amyotrophic lateral sclerosis (ALS), botulism, spina bifida, and Guillain-Barré syndrome.

Individuals with fine- or gross-motor skill limitations likely will require different types of assistive technologies at work. Fine-motor skills are used to perform tasks that involve little movements, such as typing and using a mouse. Gross-motor skills involve the big movements of the large muscles of the body, and include running and jumping.

Alternative Input Devices

Alternative input devices replace the standard keyboard and mouse on a computer or laptop. They can also replace finger pointing or a stylus on a PDA. Such devices let users with severe hand- and finger-motor impairments activate computers and PDAs in the method that's easiest for them. An alternative input device might be as simple as an ergonomic keyboard for people with arthritis. It can also be a mouse that you control with your head or foot.

Trackballs

The traditional mouse requires the user to perform three tasks at once. The user must grasp the mouse, move the mouse, and click a mouse button at the same time. By design, the trackball requires less motor control. It has separate buttons for each mouse action, including scrolling and right-click and left-click.

Some trackballs require only that you connect the cable to the computer's port. Other trackballs have supporting software to

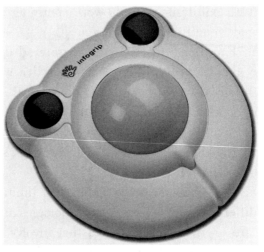

BIGtrack. *The Infogrip BIGtrack requires less fine-motor control than a standard trackball. (Source: Photo courtesy of Infogrip.)*

be installed on the computer. One great plug-and-play trackball is the three-inch BIGtrack from Infogrip; it's the largest trackball on the market.

Joysticks

Similar to trackballs, joysticks allow the user to control a computer. The difference is that you can just hold down a joystick to make it move, which can be helpful in certain situations such as drawing and playing games.

The Traxsys Roller Plus line of joysticks have six buttons that replicate a variety of mouse functions, such as right-click, double-click, and cursor speed control. They come with two different handles: a soft sponge ball or a T-bar.

TIP *To keep a joystick in place, use a mounting system. The base attaches to just about anything, including a wheelchair or table, helping to hold any device in place.*

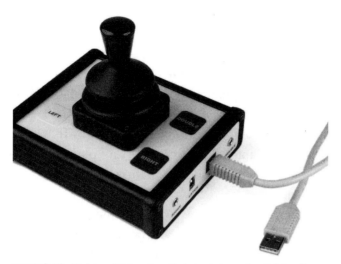

Joystick. *The Tash Joystick is a strong but simple-to-use joystick for all mouse functions. (Source: Photo courtesy of AbleNet Inc.)*

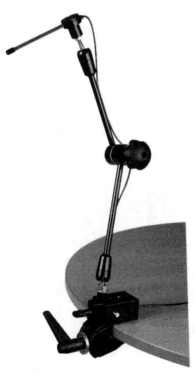

Mounting Arm. *A mounting arm, such as this one from AbleNet, attaches various switches and devices onto wheelchairs or tables. (Source: Photo courtesy of AbleNet Inc.)*

Switches

People with severe motor impairments sometimes use switches. Switches are small devices that plug into a computer. They let users control the computer with a series of movements from a foot or the head or with an eye blink or a breath.

Switches come in many forms. Many trackballs and joysticks can be "switch adapted," meaning you can plug in a switch that will let you perform an additional function, such as a mouse right-click.

There are also pneumatic switches, also called sip-and-puff switches, which have a plastic straw at the end and are activated with breath; switches that rock back and forth like a scale;

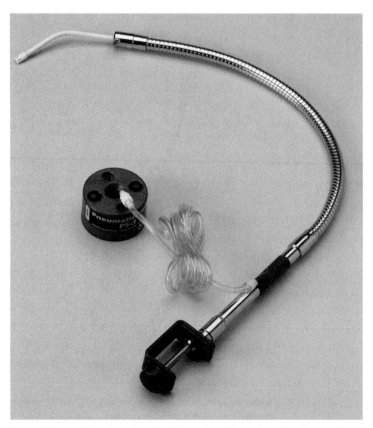

Pneumatic Switch. A sip-and-puff switch, such as this one from Prentke Romich, is activated by light blowing or sucking. (Source: Photo courtesy of Prentke Romich Co.)

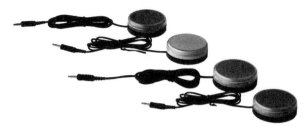

Access Switch. *A variety of switches, such as these button switches from Prentke Romich, can be used to control a computer. (Source: Photo courtesy of Prentke Romich Co.)*

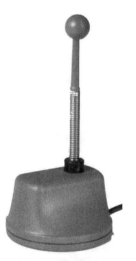

Wobble Switch. *A wobble switch, such as this one from AbleNet, can be activated from any direction by large movements. (Source: Photo courtesy of AbleNet Inc.).*

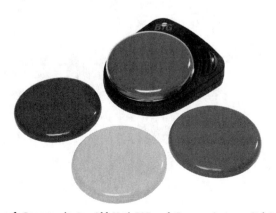

BIGmack Communicator. *AbleNet's BIGmack Communicator switch is ideal for people who need a larger target area because of motor, visual, or cognitive impairments. (Source: Photo courtesy of AbleNet Inc.)*

and wobble switches designed for large movements such as slapping. Generally, switches have a high learning curve and are often used as a last resort when other alternative input devices won't work.

The Prentke Romich Company and AbleNet sell a variety of switches.

Eye Gaze Systems

An eye gaze system is a camera that's mounted on or below a computer monitor and focused on the user's eye. The camera determines where the user is looking, and the cursor is placed at the gaze point. Mouse clicks are performed with a slow eye blink, an eye dwell, or a switch. Unfortunately, this is one of the most expensive alternative computer access products on the market, costing upward of $6,000. But the cost will often be reimbursed by insurers. LC Technologies makes the Eyegaze Edge and Eyefollower, a new device that's designed to accommodate a wider range of head motions.

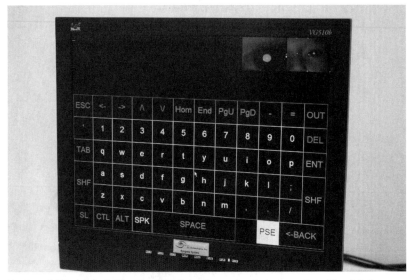

EyeGaze. LC Technologies' EyeGaze Edge helps the user control a computer with quick glances and blinking movements. (Source: Photo courtesy of LC Technologies.)

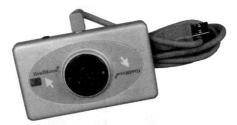

HeadMouse Extreme. *The HeadMouse Extreme from Prentke Romich replaces the standard computer mouse for people who cannot use or have limited use of their hands. (Source: Photo courtesy of Prentke Romich Co.)*

Head Tracking Systems

Less expensive than an eye gaze system, but just as good, is a head-tracking device that translates the natural movements of a user's head into directly proportional movements of the computer mouse pointer. A small camera mounted on the computer wirelessly tracks a small dot that you place on your forehead, glasses, or the rim of a hat. Most devices plug directly into a USB port, just like a mouse, and allow you to point wherever you want on the screen. Two popular choices are the TrackerPro from Madentec and the HeadMouse Extreme from Origin Instruments.

To perform a mouse click with your head, however, you'll need another configuration, such as software that lets you dwell on one spot to signal a click. For instance, you can use Madentec's TrackerPro headpointer and its MagicCursor 2000 dwell-clicking software. Then add ScreenDoors 2000, a software program for Windows that lets you select and type words from an onscreen keyboard.

Foot Control Systems

Foot switches are specially designed to be activated by the user's feet. These switches eliminate all hand mouse use and often can be programmed to perform multiple tasks with one click.

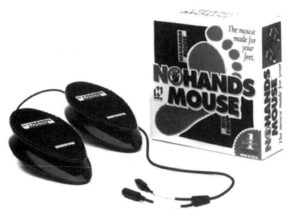

NoHands Mouse. The NoHands Mouse from Hunter Digital is designed to be activated by the user's feet and consists of two separate pedals. (Source: Photo courtesy of Hunter Digital.)

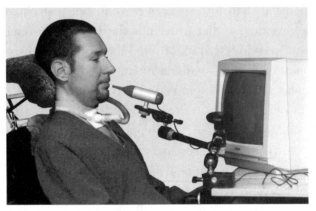

Integra Mouse. AbleNet's Integra Mouse enables the user to activate all functions of a computer mouse by mouth. (Source: Photo courtesy of AbleNet Inc.)

Mouth Control Systems

People with severe motor impairments also may choose to oper-ate their computer using their mouth. Several companies make mouth-controlled joysticks that you move with your mouth, cheek, chin, or tongue to shift the cursor wherever you want. On some models, you can perform right-click, left-click, and double-click actions with a sip-and-puff switch built into the joystick.

The Jouse2 by Compusult is a popular mouth-controlled joystick; another is AbleNet's Integra Mouse. Both devices enable the user to trigger left and right mouse clicks using very slight sucking or blowing actions.

Pen Tablets

One of the most common causes of pain today is working for long periods at a computer. People with arthritis, carpal tunnel syndrome, or repetitive stress fatigue will like the comfort of a pen tablet, an ergonomic alternative to using a mouse. Pen tablets let you work with your computer in a more relaxed position and reduce the amount of stress on your hands, wrists, and arms.

The Bamboo from Wacom is a free-moving pen and a tablet that substitutes for or complements many mouse functions. It's designed for office tasks and works with a variety of software, including Windows Vista, Microsoft Office, and Mac OS X.

If you have a severe hand or wrist injury or impairment and would like to use a pen tablet, be sure to choose a pen with a high pressure-sensitivity level for ease of use.

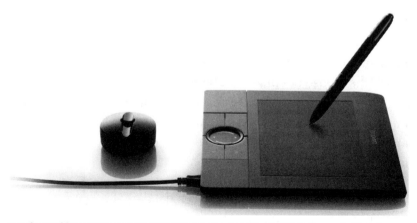

Bamboo Tablet. The Bamboo from Wacom is a pen-controlled tablet that can substitute for many mouse functions. (Source: Photo courtesy of Wacom.)

Touch Screens

Similar to the screens used on today's popular smartphones such as the Apple iPhone and the BlackBerry Storm, touch screens are a clear sheet of plastic with tiny sensors that detect pressure from either a fingertip or a pointing device. When these sensors are pressed, they perform the functions of the traditional mouse: single-click, double-click, and drag. On a computer screen they are a good alternative for someone with limited motor ability.

Touch Pads

Touch pads allow the user to move the cursor simply by dragging a fingertip across a surface. Beneath this surface is a grid-like array of sensors that detect a person's touch. The direction of the onscreen cursor is directly controlled by the movement of the user's fingertip on the surface of the touch pad. Good fine-motor control of a finger is all that is needed.

MouseKeys

MouseKeys is software that transforms a computer's numeric keypad into a directional mouse. When the software is activated, each number on the numeric keypad represents a direction in which the mouse or cursor can be moved.

For example, pressing the 6 key on the numeric keypad directs the mouse to the right. Pressing the 9 key directs the mouse up and to the right. Pressing the 1 key directs the mouse down and to the left.

Other keys on the numeric keypad perform the other functions controlled with a traditional mouse, such as single-click and drag-lock. Settings allow the acceleration and speed of the onscreen cursor to be adjusted.

You can find MouseKeys in Microsoft's Accessibility Options. On a Mac it can be found in the Universal Access settings.

Another cool application found on a Mac is Automator. Using Automator's "Watch me do" feature, you can record what you do on your Mac, save it as a workflow, and run the workflow whenever you want to perform the same series of steps.

 Apple OS X and Microsoft Windows allow you to use keyboard commands in place of a mouse. This is accomplished using the arrow or cursor keys or by pressing a specific combination of keys to activate the desired function.

Alternative Keyboards

There are also plenty of keyboard alternatives on the market. Alternative keyboards can be used by individuals with various impairments but are especially beneficial to those who experience pain and fatigue when keyboarding. Alternative keyboards come in many sizes and shapes. Many increase typing comfort, and several can be positioned to accommodate individual preferences, including negative and positive tilt adjustments.

Expanded Keyboards

Expanded keyboards are typically flat and smooth and have larger keys (e.g., one-inch square); most have a clear Mylar cover, and many are waterproof. IntelliKeys by Kurzweil Educational Systems is a popular flat keyboard that comes with customizable overlays (such as pictures) for learning.

Miniature Keyboards

Miniature keyboards are smaller than traditional QWERTY keyboards and are typically covered with a plastic membrane. Keys are closely spaced for easy access, and the keyboard surface is very sensitive to touch.

Ergonomic Keyboards

Ergonomic keyboards are designed to reduce fatigue and wrist discomfort. A contoured keyboard separates the left- and right-hand sides into two concave sections or key wells. The key wells are designed to accommodate different finger lengths, shortening the reach to distant keys and preventing harmful wrist extension.

Other keyboards are also designed with ergonomics in mind. For example, Microsoft's Natural Keyboard Elite has a wave shape that encourages natural wrist and arm alignment.

One-Handed Keyboards

One-handed keyboards and software assist individuals with no or limited use of one hand in entering data into a computer by allowing more convenient one-handed entry and control. However, some experts say that even if you have the use of only one hand you can still type on a standard keyboard.

Lilly Walters, the author of *The One Hand Typing and Keyboarding Manual*, says she learned to type up to eighty words per minute using one hand on a normal keyboard. That's faster than most people type using two hands! "It's not the violin; it's the hours of practice the violinist puts in. It's the same idea with typing," she told me.

Onscreen Keyboards

An onscreen keyboard offers an alternative to pushing keys on a real keyboard. It floats like a popup on your screen that you can operate with your mouse or alternative input device. There are onscreen keyboard software solutions for both Windows and Mac environments. ScreenDoors 2000 and Don Johnston's Discover:Screen 2.0 work with Windows; Discover Envoy works on a Mac.

ScreenDoors 2000 allows you to type directly into any application. A list of predicted words guesses what you are typing to help speed entry. Prentke Romich's WiVik comes with more than fifty different onscreen keyboards, available in twenty-two languages. The keyboards can be customized to contain any keys you want, moved anywhere on the screen, and resized. The software also includes word prediction, abbreviation expansion, and dwell selection and scanning.

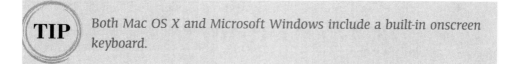

TIP Both Mac OS X and Microsoft Windows include a built-in onscreen keyboard.

StickyKeys

StickyKeys (or latch key) allows users to replicate the effect of pressing down two or more keys at once without actually doing so. Users can press one key, release it, and then press the other key or keys without having to press and hold all the keys down simultaneously.

TIP In Windows you can find StickyKeys in Accessibility Options. In Mac OS X, it can be found in the Universal Access (or Ease of Access) settings. Both operating systems also include options for slowing down the keyboard and enlarging the cursor width to allow easier handling with an alternative input device.

Software

Word Prediction

Word prediction technology attempts to guess what the user is typing. A list of words is presented to the user; selecting a number associated with the desired word causes the program to finish typing the word for the user and predict the next possible word to use.

Gus! Word Prediction software offers a list of words based on what keys the user has already pressed. As each key is pressed, the list changes accordingly to predict the current word the user is trying to enter (word completion) and the next word (word prediction). The software also offers abbreviation expansion and speech output.

EZ Keys from Words+ is another program that works with Windows to facilitate typing. It uses word completion and word prediction features to make typing easier and faster, abbreviation expansion, and can provide speech output. The distinguished astrophysicist Stephen Hawking, who is almost entirely paralyzed as a result of neuromuscular dystrophy, has limited mobility in a few fingers on his right hand and uses EZ Keys to produce and edit all of his presentations, papers, and books. EZ Keys holds up to 5,000 words and allows users to save thousands of set phrases. Hawking even uses the program to deliver live lectures.

Speech-Recognition Software

If you are unable to type or have difficulty doing so, speech-recognition software can help. Speech-recognition programs type on the computer screen the words you speak into a microphone.

To use voice-recognition software you first must train the computer to recognize your voice by reading a preset list of words. The computer makes a print of your voice for each word. This allows it to recognize your voice and accent. Each time you use it, your voice profile is resaved with any changes you made.

If it is configured properly, speech-recognition software will also provide the user with a considerable amount of hands-free control over the computer. This is a good option for those who want to limit their use of a mouse and keyboard.

Windows' built-in speech-recognition program, Windows Speech Recognition, allows you to dictate simple documents and e-mails, navigate the Internet, and command applications by saying what you see.

For more advanced communications such as dictation, however, you'll want a third-party program, such as IBM's ViaVoice or Dragon NaturallySpeaking from Nuance Communications.

NaturallySpeaking Preferred 10 has a 42,000-active-word vocabulary. You can use it to navigate your desktop and Web browser, send e-mail and instant messages by voice, and create documents across Office applications, including Word and Excel.

Similarly, Apple's built-in Speakable Items lets you control the computer using your voice instead of the keyboard. There are more than 100 speakable commands already created for the user, with no need to train the computer first. You can use Speakable Items to navigate menus and enter keyboard shortcuts, speak the names of checkboxes and radio buttons, and open, close, and switch among applications.

If you own a Mac and want to use it to create and edit documents using your voice, you'll want MacSpeech Dictate, which allows dictation, editing, formatting, and simple speech navigation within any application. Dictate frees users from the keyboard and mouse.

Headsets

While software programs usually include a headset for dictation, these aren't the most advanced devices available. Moreover, it can be difficult for users with upper-extremity issues to place a headset on their head.

Instead consider a professional-grade desktop microphone that lets you speak from anywhere in your room or office. AcousticMagic's Voice Tracker is certified for both NaturallySpeaking and MacSpeech Dictate. Voice Tracker forms a listening beam (like a searchlight) that locates and electronically steers toward the speaker. This spatial filtering reduces background noise, creating a very high signal-to-noise ratio, which results in low recognition errors, long range, and fast response.

Another option for both the PC and the Mac is the TalkFar Wireless 100 USB Voice-Recognition Microphone. This lightweight, egg-shaped microphone hangs around the neck, below the chin, for voice recognition and has a range of up to 100 feet.

Telephones

Luciano has muscular dystrophy, a condition that confines him to a wheelchair. He has severely weakened muscles, making it nearly impossible for him to lift a cell phone to his ear. Luciano uses a switch-adapted Bluetooth headset that's mounted to his wheelchair. He places his finger on a light-touch switch to start, end, and answer calls on his cell phone.

Today's speakerphones and hands-free mobile phones are great if you can still operate the buttons to activate calls. But many people with upper-extremity disabilities can't perform this simple function. There are several options available to them for telephone communication, from large-button phones to completely wireless and voice-activated dialing.

The TalkSwitch is a large-button landline phone that is switch adapted. You can plug in any type of switch to answer calls and hang up. The TalkIR Professional Infrared ECU Speakerphone from GimpGear is a full-duplex speakerphone that can be used with a switch. The TalkIR automatically adjusts its sensitivity to the strength of your voice and distance from the speakerphone.

Full-duplex technology is similar to what's found on high-end conferencing systems. A digital processor helps create clear-sounding voices without the echo effect of a regular speakerphone.

The TalkFar Wireless 100' USB Voice-Recognition Microphone also turns your computer into a wireless phone for voice over Internet protocol (VoIP) calls with Skype, ViaTalk, or Vonage, for example. You can also use it for voice recognition with Dragon NaturallySpeaking and chat programs such as Windows Live Messenger, Yahoo Messenger, Google Talk, and iChat.

Cell Phones

If you use a wheelchair, you can mount a cell phone to your chair using a special mounting arm. You can also put it on a lanyard and wear it around your neck.

Your best bet is a Bluetooth-enabled cell phone, which lets you make calls without having physically to hold the phone. The phone itself should have voice-activated on–off switching and dialing capabilities so that you can make and take calls without having to press any buttons.

However, to use Bluetooth today you must activate it on the phone or the headset. Some people can do this with their fingers, nose, elbow, tongue, or mouth.

If you can press a small button and you don't mind not having any privacy, an inexpensive option is to buy a Bluetooth speakerphone designed for use in a car and mount it to your wheelchair for hands-free calling.

People with dexterity limitations might want to consider an accessory that works with a switch to activate the Bluetooth speakerphone. SAJE Technology makes the ZoomMate, which you can use with any number of Tash switches for starting, ending, and answering calls. GimpGear makes the VoiceBT, which works with any button or sip-and-puff switch. Both products also can be used with headsets.

Mark Felling, CEO of GimpGear, which sells the VoiceBT, says, "You have the best of both worlds—a speakerphone and privacy capabilities. They're more reliable; you don't have the discomfort or health issues of having to wear it all the time on the side of your head; and you can set it next to your bed on the nightstand at night."

In addition to the ZoomMate, SAJE makes the EasyBlue, a switch-adapted Bluetooth Motorola headset that you can use with a Tash switch to activate Bluetooth without having physically to touch the phone. However, there are some disadvantages to this option. One is that it's costly: you can get the same functionality with a wired headset for much less money. Second, the headsets can be unreliable in picking up voice commands. Third, Bluetooth uses radio waves, and headsets aren't meant to be worn all day, so if you can't physically take it off and on, the headset could pose health risks.

GimpGear also has a cell phone solution for people who are completely nonvocal. The GimpGear Vocalize! Wheelchair Bluetooth Cell Phone Voice Control System allows you to answer calls, place calls, and hang up totally hands-free without pressing any buttons or having to see the phone. You simply say your magic keyword (e.g., "telephone") to activate the voice prompt. The device hooks up to your wheelchair batteries for charging and mounts underneath your seat.

The Vocalize! system can be used as a speakerphone or with a privacy headset, and is compatible with any Bluetooth-enabled cell phone that supports the hands-free profile, such as the HP iPAQ; HTC's Fuze, Touch Pro, and Touch Diamond; and the Motorola Q and XV6900. GimpGear says it will soon add support for the iPhone and iPod. There's also a portable version for people who do not use wheelchairs. The Vocalize! system costs $649 and doesn't include the phone; the portable version costs $549.

In case you didn't already know, Apple's iPod has voice control capabilities. In June 2009 Apple added voice control to the iPhone 3GS and the iTouch. You still need to press a button to activate the device, but these popular gadgets are becoming more accessible to people with physical disabilities.

> **TIP** *Under the VoiceDial Exemption Program, AT&T and SprintPCS will waive their monthly fee for voice dial services for people with any qualifying upper-extremity mobility impairment. You'll also get up to $15 worth of 411 Directory Assistance calls free each month.*

Technologies for Daily Living

A mobility disability can have a profound impact on life at home. Houses may need to be modified, cars may need to be adapted, and activities such as cooking, writing, and reading can be more difficult. There are workaround solutions for most daily living activities, though it can take some creativity and patience to figure out the best solutions for your needs.

Just look at wheelchairs. People use wheelchairs for a variety of reasons—some permanent, some temporary. The main users of wheelchairs are those who have a spinal cord injury. Other reasons for wheelchair use include fatigue from multiple sclerosis, muscle weakness from muscular dystrophy, lower-limb spasticity from cerebral palsy, and missing limbs due to amputation.

There are hundreds of wheelchairs on the market, ranging from light, manual ones to superpowered chairs that can maneuver on rough terrains. There are wheelchairs that recline, elevate, stand up, or go into a swimming pool with you. Your disability and your lifestyle will dictate the type of chair you'll want to get.

The wrong wheelchair will be totally useless, and companies sometimes charge restocking fees for returned chairs. The main things you need to know are the size and style and what type of footrest and armrest you need. Medicaid and most healthcare insurers will reimburse you the cost of a wheelchair if you qualify for one.

Manual Wheelchairs

A wheelchair is a chair mounted on large wheels. Manual wheelchairs are the lightest of the bunch. They start at around $1,000 for a basic version and weigh around thirty to forty-five pounds. Ultra-lightweight chairs can weigh less than twenty pounds. If you can use your arms, a manual wheelchair helps you maintain your mobility independence and keeps you fit, though there's a risk of shoulder injury.

Some manual wheelchair companies, such as Sunrise/Quickie, offer power-assist wheelchairs, which are manual chairs that sense your push on the hand rims and supplement your movement with some motorized power.

Newer wheelchairs, called mid-wheel-drive chairs, are extremely stable and are growing in popularity. They have six wheels and allow you to rotate in place. They also are handy for turning around in tight spaces such as an office or a minivan.

Scooters

A scooter is a wheeled cart or personal mobility vehicle with an electric motor and three or four wheels. Scooters are ideal for people who have difficulty walking for various reasons, such as fatigue or muscle weakness.

Scooters are controlled with "tillers" or handlebars, which require some upper-body strength. They're not as maneuverable as powered wheelchairs, so it's difficult to fit into small spaces and transfer surfaces such as the bed or bath. However, they're lighter than powered wheelchairs and can be broken down and stored in a car trunk or back seat.

Scooters are excellent for out-of-home use. Many public recreation areas, including Disney World, offer scooters for the convenience of customers.

Powered Wheelchairs

Powered wheelchairs, or electric wheelchairs, are more appropriate for people with significant mobility impairments. They are usually controlled with a programmable joystick, head control switch, or sip-and-puff switch. You don't need to use your arms or legs to operate a powered chair.

Chair controllers are sophisticated on a powered wheelchair, offering multiple setups for speed, acceleration, and deceleration. Remote controls allow assistants to have control over chairs, while some chairs allow electronic diagnostics over a phone line plugged into a port on the chair.

Powered chairs such as the Permobil C500 and the Levo Combi are capable of standing you up by bracing your legs while the chair motors you up on your feet.

Specialized Wheelchairs

If you haven't watched the Paralympics, you haven't seen the power of sports-designed wheelchairs. Wheelchairs for athletes have special angles and designs for increasing agility and flexibility. There are wheelchairs for basketball, tennis, and rugby. Cycling even has its own chair, the handcycle, which has a three-wheeled design and lets users pedal with their hands. For the less hard-core athlete, there are all-terrain chairs with balloon wheels for the beach and aquatic chairs for use in swimming pools.

Handcycling became an organized sport less than ten years ago, making its debut at the 2004 Summer Paralympics in Athens.

Prosthetics

South Africa's Oscar Pistorius became famous as a sprinter with no legs who runs on high-tech carbon-fiber prosthetic legs. He went on to challenge the International Association of Athletics Federations to let him compete in the Olympics against able-bodied people. He won the argument on appeal but failed to qualify. Nonetheless, he went on to take the gold medal in three events at the 2008 Paralympics in Beijing.

Upper-extremity (arm and hand) prostheses can be body powered or they can run on a battery. Electric prostheses use muscle signals to control the hook, hand, wrist, or elbow.

Lower-extremity (leg and foot) prostheses can also be conventional or computer controlled. The programmable C-leg uses computer chip technology and can be customized to work with a wearer's movement idiosyncrasies.

Prosthetics are an amazing technology: next-generation artificial limbs may one day be permanently implanted and perform much like natural limbs. This field of study becomes all the more critical when you consider that today many recipients of these prosthetics are young, active adults. It's estimated that more than 30,000 soldiers who fought in Iraq and Afghanistan have returned home with serious physical injuries. Many of these injuries are a result of homemade bombs called improvised explosive devices (IEDs).

Retired U.S. Army sergeant Juan Arredondo is just one of many recently returned veterans from Iraq. A cell phone–detonated IED that exploded in his vehicle caused extensive damage to his legs and severed his left arm just below the elbow. Sergeant Arredondo received an electric hand called the iLIMB Hand while in recovery at Brooke Army Medical Center in San Antonio.

The iLIMB Hand by Touch Bionics is an electric limb for people who have lost one or two hands or arms. The iLIMB Hand permits six separate movements, one for each digit and another for the wrist. Today Sergeant Arredondo uses his iLIMB Hand to hold a rifle or baseball, type, and grab a cup.

The Wounded Warrior Project helps injured veterans with health care and assistive technologies, including prosthetics. WWP holds a number of events across the country to raise money and awareness for veterans' needs.

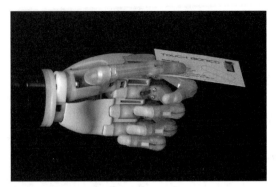

iLIMB Hand. *Touch Bionics' iLIMB Hand prosthesis imitates the true movement and accuracy of the human hand. (Source: Photo courtesy of Touch Bionics.)*

Environmental Controls

Environmental control units (ECUs) are electronic devices that let you operate home appliances and consumer electronics in one room or around the house without using your hands. Some ECUs are voice controlled; others are operated by remote controls or switches.

The user of an ECU employs spoken commands or whichever switch method he or she can most easily manage to operate a wide range of electrical devices such as lights, computers, thermostats, electric beds, televisions, DVD players, and garage doors.

Some ECUs are simple infrared remote controls for a few appliances in one room, such as the TV and the phone. Others are sophisticated systems costing thousands of dollars that will control almost everything in the house. The key is to look for a system that has excellent voice control regardless of background noise, says GimpGear's Felling.

On the low end, the Invoca Voice-Activated IR Remote for the TV comes with four simple default voice commands: power, channel up, channel down, and previous. You can program in your own voice commands to go to a specific channel using the call sign, such as ESPN or Bravo, or use macros to play a DVD, such as "Set TV to channel 3, power on speakers, turn on DVD, press play." One catch: the noise from the TV can disrupt voice control.

GimpGear's VoiceIR Infrared Environmental Voice Control System lets you start with the basics—the voice controller—and add modules and accessories that are also compatible with other ECUs as you need them. You can add a speakerphone, light dimmers, an assistance chime, or door openers. The basic package starts at $1,500.

On the high end, SAJE's Powerhouse Roommate adds voice-controlled setup to one room and costs around $2,500, while the Powerhouse Home version transforms your entire home into a voice-controlled environment, starting at around $4,500. The SiCare environmental control unit can be operated by voice, keystroke, or switch. You can control any device that is equipped with an infrared or radio receiver, including a wheelchair, TV, or powered bed. The system can also operate a SiPhone, a cordless infrared-controlled wheelchair telephone. It costs around $5,500.

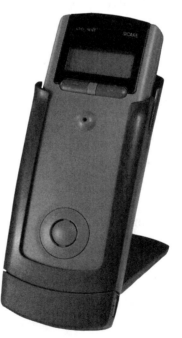

SiCare Standard. The SiCare environmental control unit lets users control numerous appliances and devices by voice alone. (Source: Photo courtesy of AbleNet Inc.)

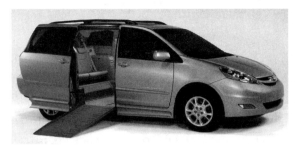

Toyota Sienna. *The Toyota Sienna wheelchair van has a roomy interior and a lightweight ramp for ease of access for wheelchair and scooter users. (Source: Photo courtesy of Toyota USA.)*

Driving

"Can you drive?" is a question asked often of people in wheelchairs. The good news is, the answer is sometimes "Yes!" There are various types of hand controls, commonly called "push–right angle–pull" controls, that move in different directions for acceleration and braking. Of course, using these requires upper-body muscles or wrist muscles.

Today, the best option for a wheelchair-using driver is an adapted minivan that is large enough to let the wheelchair slide in and out with the help of powered ramps. To this end, a van conversion company will lower the floor of vans and minivans for a better fit and design. Some popular accessible minivans include Toyota's Sienna, Chrysler's Dodge Grand Caravan, and Honda's Odyssey. GM and Ford have stopped manufacturing minivans.

Most major automobile makers have mobility programs that offer a rebate against the cost of installing adaptive equipment in a new vehicle. These programs generally reimburse $500 to $1,000 to the buyer of a new vehicle.

Even if you can't drive, you can still take advantage of adapted wheelchairs to sit in the front seat.

Exercise

There are tons of options for people with disabilities to enjoy adaptive sports. From wheelchair bowling to basketball, kayaking, skiing, and biking, all it takes is the desire to pursue your passion and, sometimes, the help of adaptive equipment. For those looking to stay fit in a less extreme fashion, consider wheelchair-friendly exercise videos such as *Chair Aerobics for Everyone* or *Chair Tai Chi.*

Another option is fitness-based videogames. The Nintendo Wii is one of the latest generation of videogame consoles. Instead of a joystick it uses a wireless controller called the Wii Remote, which contains a sensor able to detect motion and rotation. It can be used with one hand to play sports such as tennis, baseball, golf, and bowling. Thus, the Wii can be used to help people with physical disabilities exercise and stay fit. It's also used in rehab centers across the country as therapy for patients.

Reading

We're in an exciting time for audiobooks, which are digital versions of books that can be downloaded to a computer, mp3 player, or iPhone instead of held in your hands. The Audible.com and iTunes media libraries offer thousands of books for download, and if you have a qualifying print disability (e.g., you are physically unable to hold books), you can join Bookshare.org for $75 a year (or for free, if you're a K–12 or college student). Bookshare has more than 60,000 books, magazines, and periodicals, though it's skewed toward textbooks and literature.

In addition to iPods and other mp3 players, you can download books to an electronic book reader, or e-book reader. Right now, the darling of them all is the Kindle from Amazon. With a Kindle you can wirelessly download more than 350,000 titles from Amazon.com. Books cost around $10, compared with $25 for the hardcover version, and many titles have text-to-speech, so you can listen to the book instead of reading it. A newer version of the Kindle is the DX model, which has a larger, nearly ten-inch, display and is designed for reading textbooks and graphics-heavy documents. There's even a Kindle for iPhone application available in the Apple App Store. And now you can download a free Kindle app on PCs that run Windows XP, Vista, and 7. This may also be available soon on Windows mobile smartphones.

If you have a physical disability, you can control the Kindle by laying it flat on a table and pressing only the giant bar on either side to advance to the next page. However, to use more advanced controls such as accessing the menu, you'll need to be able to use buttons and a scroll wheel.

The Sony Reader is a competing device, but its lack of titles is disappointing and it has no wireless connectivity. Still, this is a market that has just begun to heat up and will only broaden in the next couple of years.

Those who like the look and feel of a good bound book can consider a mechanical book holder and page turner. The Touch Turner will hold a book in place and turn the page when the reader activates a sip-and-puff switch, for example.

There are even more advanced devices on the market that can be combined with an environmental control unit to become a voice-controlled page turner, but these cost around $4,000. You could buy 200 books at Barnes & Noble for that cost!

Home and Daily Living

Equipment that you'll likely need for adapting your home doesn't fall into the high-tech category. You can adapt your bathroom with a roll-in shower or by adding a bench with a handheld shower head. To modify rooms you may need to remove doors, and kitchens can be modified with lower cabinets and roll-under counters. If you need a lift system to get you from point A to point B, you can get one that looks like the T-bar on a ski lift.

Regular tasks such as eating and getting dressed in the morning are also more difficult with a physical disability. Solutions include small devices that aid in opening and closing buttons and zippers. The Independent Tools PocketDresser

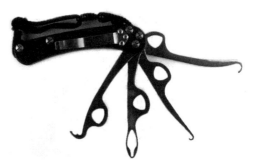

PocketDresser. The PocketDresser from Independent Tools resembles a jackknife with hooks for zippers and pulls. (Source: Photo courtesy of Independent Tools.)

is a combination buttonhook, zipper pull, and button aid that resembles a jackknife, but with hooks. Also available are modified utensils such as bendable and foam-covered forks, spoons, and knives.

Great solutions for cleaning your home are the iRobot Roomba vacuum and Scooba floor washer.

Life on wheels isn't easy, but it is doable. Just thirty years ago we didn't have curb cuts on sidewalks. Computer equipment, consumer electronics, and home appliances can already be controlled with switches and voice commands.

Voice-recognition programs are among the best assistive technologies for those who can't use a keyboard. And as the ADA continues to influence American society, we'll see more public spaces that are designed for wheelchair use. Though a myriad health and other physical challenges sometimes accompany a mobility disability, assistive technology continues to make work and life a little easier day by day.

Technologies for People with Cognitive Disabilities and Learning Disorders

6

Do not worry about your problems with mathematics.
I assure you mine are far greater.

—Albert Einstein

In the summer of 2008, *Tropic Thunder*, a movie starring Ben Stiller and Robert Downey Jr., was lambasted by the disability community. In the movie, Ben Stiller's character is an aspiring actor who makes a movie called *Simple Jack* in the hope of winning an Oscar for his efforts. Jack is referred to as a "retard."

The Special Olympics and other advocacy groups called for a boycott of the film and began a global campaign to end what they called the "R-word," asking people to pledge not to use the word to describe a developmental or intellectual disability. The movie and its aftermath also received much attention in the media, from National Public Radio to the *LA Times*. *Salon* magazine called "Never Go Full Retard"—a line from the movie—"the catchphrase of the summer."

The American Association on Intellectual and Developmental Disabilities (AAIDD) is also working to rid society of the stigma associated with an intellectual or developmental disability, having changed its name from the American Association on Mental Retardation. I have argued that the building media coverage surrounding developmental and intellectual disabilities is a good opportunity for disability advocates to educate society about these types of impairments and to bring to light some of the misunderstandings surrounding the intelligence levels and capabilities of the people who are categorized into this group.

Developmental and intellectual disabilities, like many other disabilities, lie on a spectrum. One person might have trouble learning how to read or write due to a developmental delay, while another person might have severe deficits in memory and in language and social skills that significantly affect his or her ability to hold a job, communicate, and live independently.

Developmental Disabilities

Anthony is a marketing manager at a financial services company. He's working toward his executive MBA, taking classes in the evenings and on weekends. Anthony has dyslexia and uses a scan/read program that reads aloud the textbooks, market research, and case studies he needs to prepare for marketing, finance, and statistics classes.

By definition, a developmental disability is a severe, chronic disability that begins any time from birth through age twenty-one and is expected to last for a lifetime. The effects may be cognitive, physical, or a combination of both.

A learning disability is one type of developmental disability. It involves a deficit in one's ability to process specific information or perform certain functions, including the ability to speak, listen, read, write, spell, reason, or organize time and information. However, a person with a developmental disability may not necessarily have a low IQ or other cognitive impairment but may at times experience limitations in "adaptive behaviors" such as social and practical skills.

Approximately 5.4 million Americans have developmental disabilities, according to the National Association of Councils on Developmental Disabilities (NACDD). In addition to learning disorders, types of developmental disabilities include cerebral palsy, Rett syndrome, epilepsy, autism, and Asperger's syndrome.

Autism is a brain developmental disorder characterized by impaired social interaction and communication and by restricted and repetitive behavior. These signs all manifest before a child is three years old. An autistic child may have normal or above-average intellectual capacity but atypical or less well-developed social skills. Asperger's syndrome is a related disorder known as a high-functioning form of autism.

? The National Institute of Mental Health says that autism occurs in 1 in 1,000 children in the United States. But the Centers for Disease Control and Prevention estimates that autism rates run as high as 1 in 100. For families who already have one autistic child, the odds of a second autistic child may be as high as in 1 and 20.

LD Online (ldonline.org) is a tremendous tool for parents, educators, and children who want to understand more about learning disabilities. The site, a service provided by the public television station WETA in Washington, DC, provides expert advice, resources, and questions and answers.

Assistive Technologies for Developmental Disabilities

In the workplace and classroom, individuals with developmental disabilities should be able to benefit from hardware, software, and gadgets that aid information processing. They can also benefit from modified work schedules or lesson plans and flexible approaches to completing a task.

Scan/Read Programs

Scan/read programs are a powerful technology solution for people who have difficulty with reading comprehension. These programs involve hardware (a scanner) and software (text-to-speech technology). First, a scanner is used to convert material, such as a textbook, into an electronic document. Then software is used to read aloud the text on the screen.

Scan/read programs can also highlight the text being read and allow you to alter the visual display of the printed material. You can adjust the appearance so that it's easier to read, bookmark, and add comments. Many scan/read programs also include features such as talking dictionaries and thesauruses, and most have the ability to read aloud Internet pages and e-mail.

Ray Kurzweil introduced the world's first reading machine for the blind in 1976; his company, Kurzweil Educational Systems, now also produces products for people with reading difficulties. Kurzweil 3000 (See www.kurzweiledu.com) is a popular scan/read software system for Windows and Mac environments. It uses synthesized voices coupled with features that help users access, read, and manage text. Features include text-highlighting and text-circling tools, annotations, and bookmarks. You can also use a feature called Extract that helps you create outlines, study guides, or word lists. As users type, the software speaks each letter or word so that users can recognize and correct spelling mistakes.

Dave Burns, who has dyslexia and owns an auto glass company near Rochester, New York, says that with Kurzweil 3000 he was finally able to run his business. "Suddenly, I could get through a pile of invoices that might have taken a full morning in a little more than an hour. And with much less stress," Burns said.

The Kurzweil 3000 system is expensive because it comes with a proprietary scanner and optical character recognition (OCR) software that converts print into a readable digital format. You can purchase just the text-to-speech software, called Kurzweil 3000 LearnStation, separately, but you'll still need to buy a scanner that's compatible with the system.

knfb Reading Technology's knfbReader Mobile can help those with dyslexia to read books and other printed materials. Designed for sighted individuals with reading difficulties, the device is a Nokia N82 cell phone with a five-megapixel camera loaded with character-recognition and text-to-speech software.

Text-to-Speech Software

Text-to-speech software is another way to guide those with reading comprehension difficulties. Read&Write GOLD 9 from Texthelp Systems comes with a scanning application (giving you the ability to scan printed text directly into Microsoft Word) and is especially helpful for reading and printing PDFs. It's available for both Windows and Mac OS X, and is loaded with features such as highlighting, a spellchecker, and audible dictionaries.

ClaroRead Plus from British software maker Claro Systems is a similar text-to-speech program that comes with a scanning application and is less expensive than Read&Write.

If all you need is basic help reading, say, Word documents, just use the built-in text-to-speech programs that come with Windows PCs (Windows 2000 or later) and Macs (OS X). Point your cursor to where you want the text-to-speech to start.

On a Windows computer, you can find the text-to-speech program, Narrator, in the Ease of Access Center. The Mac's text-to-speech program can be found under System Preferences, and you can alter the voice and speaking rate to your preference. Mac OS X Leopard features a new voice called Alex, a human-sounding voice that is so natural he even "breathes" when speaking long passages.

You can also read PDF files aloud by opening Adobe Reader and selecting the Read Out Loud option from the View menu.

TIP *The British Broadcasting Corporation has an excellent page on making your Windows, Mac, or Linux computer talk, at www.bbc. co.uk/accessibility.*

Dictation Software

You're loving the fact that you can listen to your computer "read" a document out loud to you. So, what if you want to create, or dictate, a document using speech? No problem. Speech-recognition software, also known as dictation software, is a reality in this day and age. Using these programs you "speak" and command the computer in order to dictate documents and e-mails, fill out forms on the Web, and open and close applications.

For around $200 you can purchase a standalone speech-recognition program such as Dragon NaturallySpeaking 10 from Nuance Communications, which works on Windows computers and on a Mac that's running Windows. The NaturallySpeaking Preferred edition is an easy-to-use program that's popular in the workplace and is considered to be highly accurate.

Windows Vista and Windows 7 have a built-in speech-recognition application that's picking up steam and garnering very good reviews. You can find Windows Speech Recognition in the control panel of your computer.

To dictate on a Mac computer you need to buy a separate application from MacSpeech called Dictate.

While dictation programs significantly reduce your need to type, they aren't designed for total hands-free control (and they make a lot of mistakes at first). The trick is to spend time training the computer to understand your voice patterns and to buy a quality USB microphone. Finally, user skill—the ability to speak clearly—will have an impact on the program.

Web and E-mail

Today's youth spend lots of time on the Web, which presents a problem for those who are unable to read or understand text. Microsoft's Narrator, Apple's VoiceOver, and text-to-speech programs can read Web pages out loud. You can also download free text-to-speech readers such as NaturalReader 7 from Natural Soft. (Learn more about screen readers in Chapter 3, "Technologies for People with Visual Disabilities.")

You can purchase third-party talking Web browsers and talking e-mail programs, such as BrowseAloud 3.0 from Texthelp and QualiWEB Pro by QualiLife.

Some U.S. government agencies, organizations, and even a few corporations have outfitted their external Web sites with BrowseAloud; it's free for the consumer, while the Web site owners pay a yearly charge to use the software.

And did you know that you can also use built-in voice-recognition programs for sending e-mails instead of typing them? A neat solution, Web Trek Connect by AbleLink, lets you record messages using your computer's microphone and sends them through Microsoft Outlook or Hotmail.

Electronic Helpers

Electronic spellers and talking dictionaries are also helpful tools for people with reading disabilities. Franklin makes handheld devices that look like PDAs and provide a variety of speaking dictionaries, including collegiate, children's, and Spanish–English dictionaries. The company also sells devices with thesauruses, spelling checkers, and grammar guides.

Another neat tool is a reading pen, a portable pen-shaped scanner that holds an audible dictionary and thesaurus. The pen scans words on a page and defines and pronounces them aloud. The Readingpen Advanced Edition from Wizcom Technologies contains more than 600,000 words, which are enlarged on the Readingpen's display. The words and definitions are spoken aloud using text-to-speech technology. There's also a basic versions for students in grades K through 12.

Recently, gadget lovers have been over the moon about Livescribe's Pulse Pen, a ballpoint pen loaded with a digital recorder. The Pulse captures handwritten notes and simultaneously records, say, a teacher's lecture, and likes the audio to your notes. By simply tapping on the notes with the smartpen, you can hear the conversation play back. All of this information can

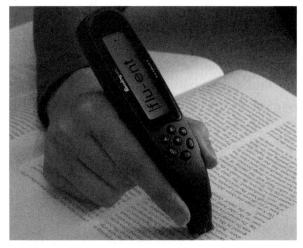

Readingpen. *The Readingpen from Wizcom Technologies. (Source: Photo courtesy of Wizcom Technologies.)*

be uploaded to a PC or Mac. The only catch is that you have to buy special notepaper to make the whole system work.

A more advanced device is Key to Access by Premier Assistive Technology. It's a small, portable USB player (you can carry it on your keychain) that holds up to ten programs, including the company's proprietary scan/read software, called Scan and Read Pro, a talking word processor, a PDF reader, tools for reading e-mails and Web pages, word prediction software, a talking dictionary and calculator, and more.

On the Internet, you can check out online dictionary and thesaurus Web sites that include audio pronunciations, such as Microsoft's Encarta, Merriam-Webster, and the Free Dictionary by Farlex, which includes lists of idioms and abbreviations and even language translators.

Another option is to use your computer's built-in dictionary and thesaurus or to download third-party software onto your computer. Merriam-Webster's *Collegiate Dictionary and Thesaurus*, Microsoft's *Encarta Right-Click Dictionary*, and the *Cambridge Advanced Learner's Dictionary* are good. Cambridge has even made its dictionary available for download on the iPhone and iTouch. Paragon Software offers its talking dictionary for the iPhone, too.

Books and Audiobooks

Reading doesn't have to be difficult, and out of the classroom and office you can read for fun with audiobooks and electronic book readers.

Looking for a book that just appeared on the *New York Times* Bestseller List? Buy the CD at a bookstore or rent it at your local library. You can also download a digital book from Audible.com or iTunes and listen to it on an mp3 player such as an iPod.

A newer invention on the market is the e-book reader, which gives you a digital version of a book. Amazon makes an e-book reader called the Kindle in two different sizes: with 6-inch and 9.7-inch displays (the latter a good choice for textbooks). You can download any of Amazon's more than 350,000 books for the Kindle wirelessly and, in most cases, use the audio feature to listen to the books out loud. (At the time of writing, Amazon is facing pressure from publishers to turn off the audio feature due to copyright issues.) Books formatted for the Kindle can also be read on the iPhone and iTouch.

Don't have a Kindle? Many smartphones, including the BlackBerry Curve, Palm Treo, and Motorola Q, let you download books by installing free e-book readers on your device. While you can't listen to these books out loud, many readers, including Mobipocket for the BlackBerry, let you annotate, bookmark, and highlight any part of an e-book.

If you have a qualifying learning disability, you can download books and magazines in audio versions from Bookshare.org for a small membership fee (free for qualifying students). One advantage of using Bookshare is that books come in DAISY (Digital Accessible Information System) format, which lets you bookmark pages and search for words—a great tool for schoolwork. Bookshare also gives students a complimentary copy of e-book software for reading DAISY books.

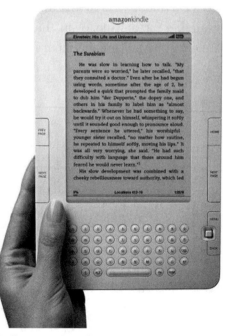

Kindle. Amazon's Kindle e-book reader lets you wirelessly download books from its audiobooks library. (Source: Photo courtesy of Amazon.)

Writing and Spelling

People who have difficulties with written language have a condition known as dysgraphia. These individuals struggle with handwriting, spelling, and composition, and will benefit from voice-recognition and text-to-speech software.

Another great technology—and a lifesaver for those with dysgraphia—is word-processing software, such as Microsoft Word, that not only includes a spellchecker but also can "say" what a person has typed when text-to-speech is turned on.

Some standalone word-processing programs also include talking dictionaries. Don Johnston's Write:OutLoud is a talking word processor and writing program aimed at students. It includes a homonym finder for students who confuse the spellings of words that sound alike, such as "blew" and "blue." It also has a talking dictionary and a feature for creating bibliographies.

Another kind of assistive technology that helps struggling writers and spellers is word prediction software. Such programs use speech output; they anticipate the word you're looking to type and provide a list of possibilities.

They also provide word completion and abbreviation expansion, as well as a spellchecker. For example, using Gus! Word Prediction by Gus Communications, you can type "GM" and up will pop "Good Morning." Don Johnston makes a similar program called Co:Writer.

And not to be outdone, Mac OS X Leopard even has a word completion program. After typing a few characters, simply press the Escape key. Leopard displays a list of words beginning with the characters you have typed.

Math and Numbers

A person with a math disability, sometimes called dyscalculia, has trouble learning and manipulating numbers. It is difficult for these individuals to understand math concepts, memorize math facts, and understand how math problems are organized on a page. They may also have difficulty with time and measurements.

Several vendors make mathematics software programs that can be customized for learning and teaching math concepts at different levels. Design Science makes MathType, and IntelliTools makes Classroom Suite 4 as well as MathPad Plus for learning fractions and decimals. Likewise, DynaVox Mayer-Johnson's Boardmaker can be customized for math classes.

For more practical math, Money Skills by Marblesoft reinforces how to use money properly. RJ Cooper makes Calculator Talk 'n Scan, an onscreen calculator with text-to-speech. Premier Assistive Technology makes a suite of math learning software tools, including Talking Calculator and Talking Checkbook. MaxiAids sells a variety of talking calculators and alarm clocks.

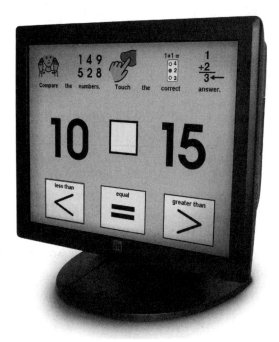

Boardmaker for Math. DynaVox's Boardmaker for Math is a popular program in classroom settings for assisting students with learning mathematical reasoning and numbers. (Source: Photo courtesy of DynaVox Mayer-Johnson, Pittsburgh, PA [866-DYNAVOX].)

Speech and Communication

Also known as dysphasia, a speech disorder or speech comprehension disorder ranges from complete absence of speech to difficulty in naming a few objects. Individuals with mild speech disorders can benefit from text-to-speech software such as ClaroRead Plus and Read&Write GOLD 9. Both programs will speak aloud any text, as will the built-in speech-recognition engines in Windows and Mac OS X. Students and professionals may find it helpful to use text-to-speech software when giving a presentation.

For more severe speech disorders, speech generator devices and other communications aids can help. You can purchase devices (about the size of a netbook) that are preloaded with speech software or use an existing Pocket PC or smartphone and install the software yourself.

Gus Communications makes MobileTTS, which equips the iPhone or BlackBerry with a text-to-speech application. You can read more about these solutions in Chapter 7, "Technologies for People with Communications Disabilities."

Personal Digital Assistants

PDAs and smartphones are also great resources for those who have difficulty managing their time and remembering schedules or routines. For example, a PDA such as an iPhone or BlackBerry can be used to set reminders for important events and to create "to-do" lists and populate a calendar.

Intellectual Disabilities

Devin Max has an intellectual disability as a result of a genetic condition. His IQ is 50. He needs help with some daily tasks, such as making his lunch and remembering the bus schedule to get to work. Devin Max uses a PDA that provides step-by-step visual and verbal instructions for these tasks, enabling him to live independently without twenty-four-hour care.

An intellectual disability differs from a developmental disability. An intellectual disability involves significant limitations in overall intellectual functioning and is generally categorized as having an IQ of 70 or below.

An intellectual disability may occur from a congenital disorder or as the result of a traumatic event such as brain injury or lead poisoning, or it may be brought about by the onset of a dementing condition such as Alzheimer's disease. Today, there are 7–8 million Americans with an intellectual disability, according to the AAIDD, and the term "intellectual disability" is replacing the term "mental retardation."

People with intellectual or developmental disabilities can benefit from a combination of home-help aids, education, training, medicine, therapy, and, of course, assistive technology. Some individuals can take jobs where they're able to master certain intellectual tasks and use assistive technology as needed.

Through behavioral training and role-playing classes, these individuals can also learn how to master social and practical skills such as how to get dressed for work or how to pay for coffee. These classes are provided through state rehabilitation agencies as well as by national disability organizations such as Easter Seals or the Arc of the United States.

Assistive Technologies for Intellectual Disabilities

Individuals with intellectual disabilities can benefit from a variety of assistive technologies discussed in Chapters 5 and 7 of this book.

Personal Digital Assistants

Computer users will appreciate portable devices that make their work and home life easier for them and their caregivers. A hand-held PDA is a good solution.

A PDA can use pictures and audio messages to help people with intellectual disabilities perform daily tasks and make decisions more independently. For example, with a Pocket PC that runs on Windows Mobile, an individual can use AbleLink Technologies' family of software, which includes Pocket Coach, a program that provides verbal prompting for step-by-step tasks and helps users make appropriate decisions. Pocket Endeavor is a great tool for work "to-do" lists. And Pocket ACE helps those with difficulty remembering people's names to store photos and other information about them onscreen.

Other AbleLink programs include Schedule Assistant, which helps individuals remember appointments, daily routines, and schedules, and Visual Assistant, which allows caregivers to incorporate pictures of instructional tasks. For example, a caregiver can record instructions while showing step-by-step pictures for preparing a salad.

AbleLink's software can be used in a desktop environment if individuals don't need a PDA.

> *e-Buddies is an e-mail pen pal program that pairs a person with an intellectual disability in a one-to-one e-mail friendship with a peer volunteer who does not have an intellectual disability. e-Buddies (www. ebuddies.org) is a program of Best Buddies, a nonprofit dedicated to enhancing the lives of people with and without intellectual disabilities.*

Keyboards

To aid computer access, Cambium Learning (the parent of Kurzweil Educational Systems) makes IntelliKeys, a keyboard with a

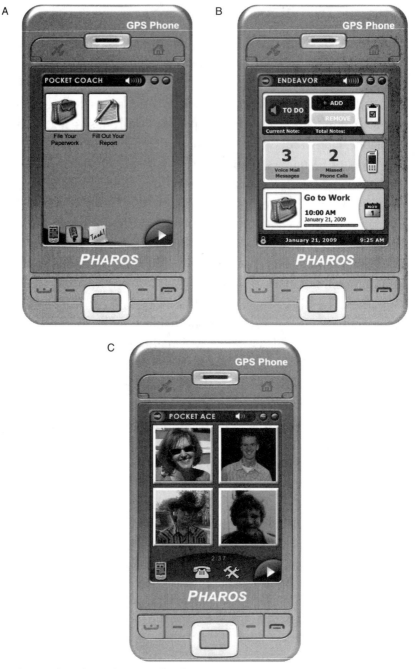

Pocket Coach, Pocket Endeavor, and Pocket ACE. Pocket Coach (A), Pocket Endeavor (B), and Pocket ACE (C) from AbleLink are designed to help users with intellectual disabilities function more independently in the workplace and at home. (*Source: Photos courtesy of AbleLink Technologies.*)

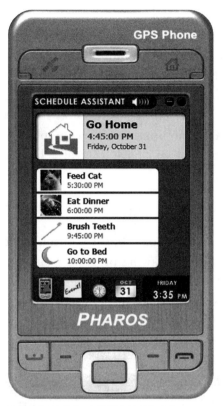

Schedule Assistant. AbleLink's Schedule
Assistant helps users remember daily routines
and schedules. (Source: Photo courtesy of AbleLink
Technologies.)

changing face. It's a USB-connected device onto which you can slide a variety of overlays, or alternative keyboard faces. Overlay content can include words, phrases, and macros, as well as letters, numbers, and the functions of the standard keyboard. The areas on the keyboard can be labeled with icons, images, and tactile representations. The company's Overlay Maker lets you make your own keyboard. For example, a user who wants to write e-mails to friends might use an overlay that includes words and descriptions about his family, hometown, and pets.

REACH Interface Author 5 is a Windows-compatible onscreen keyboard that comes with a vast assortment of assistive technology. It helps people use a computer more easily and augments their speech if needed.

REACH 5 serves as a platform for the REACH Sound-It-Out Phonetic Keyboard, on which users can type a word by selecting the sounds in the word instead of the letters. REACH 5 features 120 different keyboards with dozens of possible words or message combinations. For example, a user might generate the message "May I have a bagel?" by clicking on a picture of a bagel.

Communications Boards

For caregivers, DynaVox Mayer-Johnson's Boardmaker for Windows or Mac is a drawing program combined with a graphics database that includes 4,500 picture communication symbols for creating symbol-based living skills materials. Users can import photos of people performing step-by-step activities such as

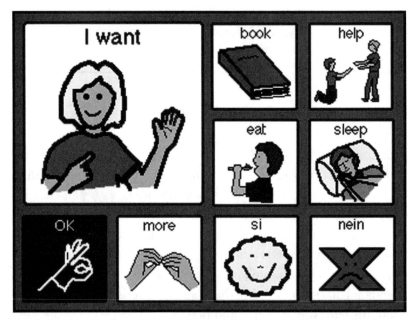

Boardmaker. DynaVox's Boardmaker is a database of graphic communication symbols that can be searched on the computer and is helpful for caregivers of augmented communicators. (Source: Photo courtesy of DynaVox Mayer-Johnson, Pittsburgh, PA [866-DYNAVOX].)

personal hygiene/grooming, toileting, meal preparation, and daily routines. Boardmaker also works well in classroom settings.

Developmental and intellectual disabilities are the most complex of all disabilities, because many disorders involve the brain and cognitive functions—an area of research that hasn't been fully figured out. It has only been in the past year or so, for instance, that scientists have discovered a handful of genes that may cause autism. As this field of research expands, more assistive technologies will be developed for those with these impairments.

Technologies for People with Communications Disabilities

7

> *A person's character is revealed by their speech.*
> —Greek proverb

Here's something I bet you didn't know. Daffy Duck and Bugs Bunny and many of their Looney Tunes friends got their quirky voices from actor Mel Blanc, who was known for giving speech impediments or otherwise quirky accents to the characters he voiced.

Both Bugs Bunny and Sylvester the Cat have noticeable lisps. Sylvester's nemesis, Tweety Bird, has a speech impediment and is known to exclaim, "I tawt I taw a puddy tat!"

Likewise, Elmer Fudd has a speech sound disorder, prompting his classic line, "Be vewy vewy quiet, I'm hunting wabbit!" And, of course, who can forget Porky Pig's famous stutter at the end of every Looney Tunes program: "Th-th-th-that's all folks!"

Developmental Speech and Language Disorders

Communication is the essence of life and is an integral part of our success in life. Communication is what enables us to articulate our thoughts and get our point across clearly to other people, whether it's our boss, our doctor, or our family.

Being unable to speak is an obstacle, but with assistive technology you can still find ways to communicate with co-workers, family, and friends. Many of the ways in which we communicate do not involve our vocal cords; for example, we use body language, and we also use technology, such as e-mail and instant messaging programs, to talk to others.

Those who have difficulty with speech or language may have a communication disability or disorder. There are many different kinds of communication disabilities; some are related to development, while others are psychological in nature. Many people affected by a communication disorder have lost some or all of their oral motor skills as a result of another disability or medical condition.

Dolores, who has difficulty with stuttering, gets very nervous when she goes on job interviews. She wears a fluency device in her ear that provides her with auditory feedback of her words, giving her more confidence and calmness to speak about her skills and qualifications.

A communications disability that begins at a young age is often called a developmental speech or language disorder. Such disabilities include having a lisp, stuttering, and cluttering. A lisp causes someone to have difficulty pronouncing sibilant letters such as "s" and "z," which tend to emerge with a "th" sound. For example, the words "salad" and "pizza" might sound more like "thalad" and "pitha."

Someone who stutters has difficulty with the flow of speech, which is constantly interrupted by involuntary repetitions of sounds, syllables, words, or phrases—or even by silent pauses during which the stutterer is unable to produce any sound at all.

Cluttering, also called tachyphemia, is characterized by speech that is difficult for listeners to understand due to a person's rapid speaking rate, erratic rhythm, or poor syntax or grammar. While stuttering is a speech disorder, cluttering is a language disorder. A stutterer knows what he wants to say but can't say it; a clutterer can say what she is thinking, but her thinking becomes disorganized during speech.

The actor James Earl Jones was virtually mute as a child. With the help of his high school English teacher he overcame his stuttering by reading Shakespeare out loud. He went on to become a Shakespearean actor and is famous for his role in the Star Wars films, in which he voiced the character Darth Vader.

Developmental disorders such as autism can also affect speech or language. As with other speech disorders, the problem may be physiological, or it may be psychological, where the speech impediment emerged as a reaction to stress or trauma.

While speech therapy is a popular course of treatment, some individuals have had success with assistive technologies that help train them to speak accurately. One treatment for stutterers is a fluency device, also known as an antistuttering device. It looks and is worn like a hearing aid and provides auditory feedback to a person who stutters throughout the day. It can be worn during business meetings and telephone calls and in day-to-day conversations.

Rather than amplify sound, fluency devices use altered feedback to create what's called a "chorale effect"—the phenomenon that occurs when people who stutter can actually speak or sing in unison with others. When stutterers wear a fluency device and speak, their words are digitally replayed in their ear with a very slight delay and frequency modification. As a result, the brain perceives them as speaking in unison with another person, which causes the chorale effect.

Fluency devices can help control speech fluency, slow down speech rate, and increase confidence. Many stutterers have had success in either reducing or eliminating their stuttering. However, fluency devices are not a cure; there is no cure for stuttering.

You can buy fluency devices through speech language pathologists. The SpeechEasy, from the Janus Development Group, is a fluency device that was featured on *Oprah* in 2007. There are several models to choose from, just as with hearing aids, from behind-the-ear to completely in-canal ones. They cost between $4,000 and $5,000.

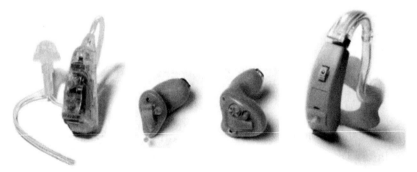

SpeechEasy. *The Janus Development Group makes a variety of models of its fluency device, the SpeechEasy. (Source: Photo courtesy of Janus Development.)*

A similar in-the-ear device is the Fluency Master, developed by the National Association for Speech Fluency. Casa Futura Technologies makes the SmallTalk, which is a "box" that you carry in your purse or pocket. It's used with a Bluetooth wireless headset or earpiece with a microphone and can be hooked directly into a telephone.

A good alternative to in-the-ear devices is a software program that you use with headphones and a microphone for a similar auditory experience. While this solution isn't as inconspicuous as an in-the-ear device, it's less expensive and can provide a good training experience at home, work, or school. Since these programs are used with Bluetooth wireless headphones, most people will think you're on the phone or listening to music on your computer.

The DAF/FAF (delayed auditory feedback/frequency altered feedback) Assistant from ArtefactSoft can be used on a computer or laptop, and the Pocket DAF/FAF Assistant can be used on a Windows Mobile Pocket PC.

There's also a DAF/FAF Assistant for the iPhone (and iTouch) that can be downloaded from either iTunes or Artefact's Web site (www.artefactsoft.com). A seven-day free trial is available.

> **TIP** For the DAF/FAF Assistant for the iPhone, Artefact recommends using Apple headphones with remote and microphone, available in the Apple Store.

Other Speech Disorders

Some speech and language impairments resemble stuttering and cluttering but are caused by disabilities and medical conditions. Dysarthria and aphasia are oral motor disorders caused by a neurological injury, such as a stroke or brain injury, or a neuromuscular disorder, such as cerebral palsy or Parkinson's disease. Dysarthria can cause slow, distorted, or slurred speech, while people with aphasia may be able to speak but not write, or vice versa.

Apraxia is a disorder that may result from a stroke or be developmental in nature. It causes someone to produce inconsistent speech sounds and rearrange words—saying "motato" instead of "tomato," for instance.

Autism, a brain developmental disorder, is characterized by impaired social interaction and communication. Children with autism may be verbal or nonverbal. About a third to a half of people with autism do not develop enough natural speech to meet their daily communication needs. This may be noticeable from the first year of life and can include delayed onset of babbling and other verbal expressions.

People who have autism may also have a condition called echolalia that causes the immediate repetition of a word or phrase. Echolalia is also sometimes present in Tourette's syndrome, aphasia, Asperger's syndrome, and Alzheimer's disease.

Augmentative and Alternative Communication

Augmentative and alternative communication, or AAC, is any nonverbal form of communication. We all use AAC to supplement our verbal communication—through our eye movements and facial gestures, for example. However, some people need extra assistance, and this is where AAC products and devices come into play.

AAC devices range from low-tech, print-based communication boards to high-tech, speech-generating devices. There are dozens of models, from dozens of manufacturers, on the market, varying greatly in price, features, and size.

Communication Boards

Communication boards are displays that help people communicate. "No-tech" boards are simple printed pages with pictures and symbols.

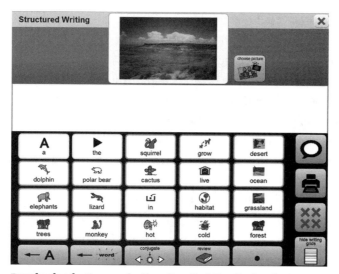

Boardmaker for Communications. *DynaVox's Boardmaker Plus is a software program that helps students and others create interactive picture boards for communicating. (Source: Photo courtesy of DynaVox Mayer-Johnson, Pittsburgh, PA [866-DYNAVOX].)*

High-tech boards are made using board-making software such as Boardmaker from DynaVox Mayer-Johnson, which provides more than 100 board templates and has a database of 4,500 pictures and symbols to help the user create and print a customized board. A more feature-rich program, Boardmaker Plus, lets users create onscreen interactive boards with the addition of sounds, voices, and animation.

Speech-Generating Devices

Devices that provide voice output are called speech-generating devices. These devices look like touch tablets equipped with a processor, memory, and high-quality speakers. The display screen is designed to let communicators select words, phrases, or pictures to be spoken aloud.

Some speech-generating devices use digitized speech that has been prerecorded by a real person (a speech therapist or caretaker) and sounds very natural. However, digitized devices do not allow a person to create new messages independently or have "live" conversations as their needs dictate. These devices are good for school-age children who are too young to master a more complex communications system.

One benefit of these devices is that they're fun for young people to use: children like the ability to press pictures and single words to help them communicate.

The Great Talking Box Company makes the EasyTalk, an easy-to-use box with twenty picture buttons that can be customized for the user. Words+ sells the MessageMate, which is about the size of an iTouch.

AbleNet makes a compact digital speech gadget that's designed to grow up with its young user. The SuperTalker starts as a single-message communicator for early communicators and can the interface be configured into a two-, four-, or eight-message communicator with interchangeable words and phrases as the user becomes a more mature communicator.

Synthesized speech devices are a far more popular choice among AAC users because they use technology to translate a

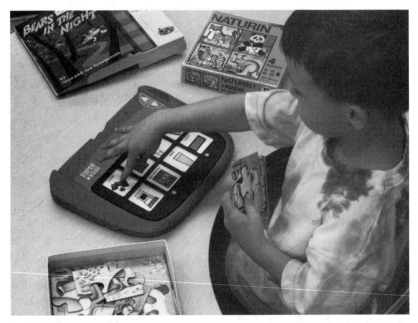

SuperTalker. AbleNet's SuperTalker is a speech-generating device that's designed to grow with users as they age and advance their vocabulary. (Source: Photo courtesy of AbleNet Inc.)

user's input into "live" speech. Today there are many high-quality-sounding voice programs on the market, including NeoSpeech and AT&T Natural Voices, that offer numerous male and female voices in multiple languages.

Some AAC devices perform double or even triple duty, functioning as a communications device, a laptop for Web browsing, e-mail, and word processing, and an environmental control unit for the television, wireless Internet, and telephone.

The most important decision is figuring out which one will work best for the user's cognitive and physical abilities. For example, some people prefer pictures, while others prefer typing words. Some users may need a device that can be mounted to a wheelchair and has multiple access methods:

- Touch: Selection is made on contact with or on release of the touch screen with a finger or stylus
- Scanning: The device automatically highlights areas of the screen in a pattern until the user selects the desired object; selection can be accomplished using a switch or other device
- Auditory scanning: The user listens as the device speaks and then hits a switch when a desired message is heard
- Morse code: the user inputs Morse code using one or two switches, with visual and audio feedback
- Head tracking: The user controls the cursor using small head or neck movements with a device atop the computer monitor that transmits a signal and tracks a small reflector dot placed on the user's head or eyeglasses.
- Eye tracking: The user controls the cursor and makes selections by gazing or blinking at the computer screen, while a camera mounted atop the computer monitor determines the gaze point.

The Freedom LITE from Words+ is a five-pound laptop with an Intel processor; it can be preloaded with Windows to make it a full computer. Features include built-in wireless capability; a DVD/CD-RW drive that allows CD-ROMs to be rewritten; and

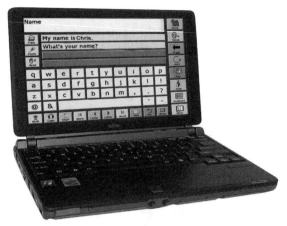

Freedom LITE. *The Freedom LITE by Words+ is a laptop-based AAC device that works well in workplace settings. (Source: Photo courtesy of Words+.)*

EZ Keys, a program that works with Windows to facilitate typing, with features such as word prediction.

British theoretical physicist Stephen Hawking, who is disabled by neuromuscular dystrophy and cannot speak, uses a Freedom computer to give presentations and lectures and to communicate with his students and colleagues. He once joked that he had everything he needed, except that the synthesized voice sounded "too American." (Engineers have since provided him with a more British-sounding inflection.)

TIP *Medicare, Medicaid, and private insurance often fund AAC devices under the speech-generating device (SGD) category. However, they will fund only the portion that's "dedicated" to speech, not the extras.*

The DynaVox V and Vmax from DynaVox Mayer-Johnson are sleek, powerful tablets with crisp display screens. They come in five colors (black, blue, green, pink, and silver) and work with a range of ages, cognitive abilities, and skill levels. They cost around $7,500.

The DynaVox V has an eight-inch screen, and the Vmax has a twelve-inch screen. They can also be used as a Windows computer. Features include 25,000 premade pages for selecting words,

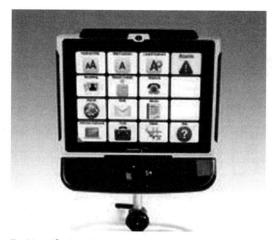

EyeMax. *The DynaVox EyeMax system allows augmented communicators to access their Vmax with a simple blink or by dwelling on a desired area of the screen. (Source: Photo courtesy of DynaVox Mayer-Johnson, Pittsburgh, PA [866-DYNAVOX].)*

pictures, or phrases, a phrase prediction program, a dictionary, a media player, and an e-book reader.

For those with motor impairments, both systems can be accessed through any of nine methods, including touch, scanning, Morse code, and eye tracking. DynaVox's new eye-tracking accessory, EyeMax, lets users access the Vmax with a simple blink or by dwelling on a desired area of the screen.

DynaVox isn't the only company with eye-controlled technology. Prentke Romich makes the ECO, a large-screen AAC speech generator that can also be configured as a full computer and environmental control unit. The ECO can be operated with ECOpoint, an eye-gazing technology introduced in 2009.

RJ Cooper & Associates, a small manufacturer based in California, makes a simpler speech generator that sells at about half the price of a Vmax. The Super Auggie is a slate PC that's about the size of a piece of paper. It has a twelve-inch display screen and runs Windows software and Speaking Dynamically Pro.

Two other devices are worth a mention. Gus Communications' Gus! Communicator U8 and the TuffTalker Convertible from Words+ can be converted from a touch-screen tablet to a laptop—and back again—with a twist of the wrist.

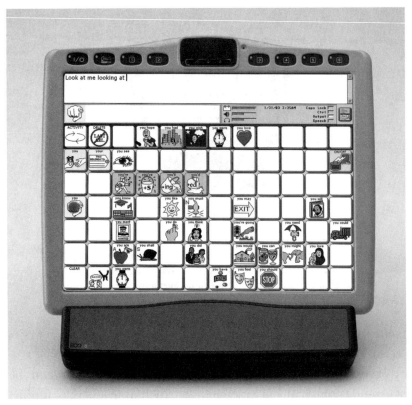

ECOpoint. ECOpoint is an eye-gazing technology for use with the Prentke Romich ECO speech generator system. (Source: Photo courtesy of Prentke Romich Co.)

Handheld AAC Devices

Handheld AAC devices have great potential for professionals and for users who are always on the go. They can be used in a car, on an airplane, and at the dinner table.

Generally about six-inches wide (smaller than a Kindle) these are excellent choices if you're able to use a small handheld computer and have enough finger and hand control to make selections from a screen with your finger, a pen, or a stylus.

While handhelds don't have as much power as full-blown computer systems, many include sophisticated voice options, lots of memory, wireless Internet, and Windows Mobile, which includes Microsoft Office and Internet Explorer.

The Xpress is a handheld AAC device from DynaVox Mayer-Johnson. It's a small, lightweight PDA that features the same touch screen as an iPhone or BlackBerry storm. This device is fine for someone who has fairly good motor control. However, if you lack the dexterity to use your fingers to find words and phrases, the Xpress might not work for you.

The Gus! Pocket Communicator works with a pocket PC, which is a personal digital assistant that runs on Windows Mobile, such as the HP iPaq. It has a four-inch screen, comes loaded with NeoSpeech, a high-quality speech generator, and includes more than 5,000 communication symbols. Users who have some speech capabilities will appreciate the ability to record messages in their own voice.

The Say-It! SAM Communicator from Words+ runs on Windows Mobile. It is a touch-screen gadget that comes in seven colors. It costs between $3,000 and $3,500, depending on which voice option you choose.

RJ Cooper's handheld Mini Auggie is built from an HP iPaq pocket PC. As with many of its products, RJ Cooper prices the Mini Auggie aggressively, though some functions may be limited.

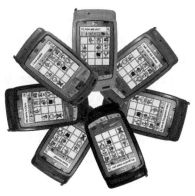

Say-It! SAM Communicator. *The Say-It! SAM Communicator from Words+ provides picture- and text-based communication in a lightweight device. (Source: Photo courtesy of Words+.)*

AAC Software

Companies that make AAC devices often also make standalone AAC software designed to work with your existing desktop, laptop, or PDA to help you communicate. Buying the software works out less expensive than buying a new device.

Your own computer supplies the speech output, or you can purchase add-on text-to-speech engines such as NeoSpeech, DECtalk, or AT&T Natural Voices.

DynaVox Mayer-Johnson's Boardmaker with Speaking Dynamically Pro, or SD Pro, is a "talking" word- and picture-processing program that has features similar to those of Boardmaker Plus. SD Pro includes word prediction, abbreviation expansion, and the ability to talk in human-sounding voices without having to purchase a separate text-to-speech engine.

TIP *Many AAC companies let you download free, thirty-day trial versions of their software from their Web sites.*

AAC users give rave reviews about The Grid 2 by Sensory Software. The Grid system uses symbol communication to build sentences and speak phrases. While the program comes with a readymade set of vocabularies, it's highly customizable—and the display can even be re-created from scratch.

Like many applications, Talking Screen by Words+ has an advanced word prediction program that lets you modify words and add new words to your personal vocabulary.

Gus Communications' SpeechPRO lets you customize the program and input information any way you want, and it works with a variety of switches, making it a good choice for those with dexterity or motor issues.

AAC on Your iPhone

Not to be outdone, the BlackBerry and iPhone are getting into the synthesized speech business. Text-to-speech applications for smartphones are now available for download from the iTunes library, effectively turning these smartphones into pocket AAC devices.

One such application is Proloquo2Go from AssistiveWare, which was recently profiled in *USA Today*. J. W. Clark, a seven-year-old boy with autism, downloaded Proloquo2Go onto an iTouch and used it to "talk" to family and friends by touching icons to express phrases, comments, or questions. Clark also uses the iTouch to communicate with his service dog (using the device's speakers). This is a good solution for kids and teens who want to be able to use a cool, mainstream device to help them talk. Proloquo2go costs $189 plus the cost of an iPhone or iTouch.

Gus Communications makes similar software. MobileTTS works on both the iPhone and the iTouch, as well as the BlackBerry Curve and Storm. This software is expensive, at around $700 (which doesn't include the phone), but it is the only solution available for BlackBerry users.

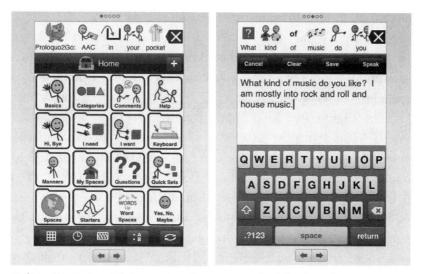

Proloquo2Go. *Proloquo2Go is a popular software program that helps those who cannot communicate with their family and friends.*

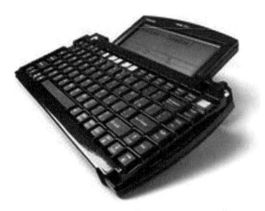

DynaWrite. *The DynaWrite from DynaVox is a talking word processor that offers an alternative to a speech-generating device. (Source: Photo courtesy of DynaVox Mayer-Johnson, Pittsburgh, PA [866-DYNAVOX].)*

Talking Word Processors

Need AAC but don't like fancy computers? There are a few communications products on the market that will work for you. These products resemble the word-processing machines that were popular in the early 1990s, before laptops were invented—except, of course, that these versions are speech enabled.

The DynaWrite from DynaVox is ideal for individuals who want the familiarity of a simple keyboard. It has a large display, with text size up to seventy-two points. Features include word prediction, a spellchecker, and word morphology (for providing correct word form).

The Lightwriter, also from DynaVox, has fewer features but boasts a dual display to enable face-to-face conversation: one screen faces the talker and the other screen faces the listener. And one more gadget that has lit up the chat rooms on tech Web sites is Livescribe's Pulse Pen. This ballpoint smartpen has a computer inside of it that can record spoken words and play them back by simply pressing the pen onto the page. This is a great, inexpensive solution for the classroom; for example, a parent or teacher can record lesson vernacular in advance so that a nonspeaking student can participate verbally along with classmates.

Telephones

Most augmented communicators talk on the telephone by positioning the phone's receiver near their device. This becomes an even handier option when they are using a handheld AAC device such as the Palm or the iPhone.

For private conversations, you can hook up your AAC device to accessories such as PhoneIT from DynaVox, which connects a standard telephone landline to your DynaVox device.

Advances in technology mean that you can also use computers to have conversations with colleagues, family, and friends. Instant messaging programs such as iChat, AIM, and Skype are a good bet for two-way conversations with friends and family using a combination of speech, text, and video.

You can also try text-to-speech programs that will turn your typed words into speech. JITA Technologies' Speech Assistant is a telephone interface that sends text-to-speech audio from a computer, PDA, or speech-generating device directly into a cordless or cell phone. This allows people with speech impairments to make and receive phone calls over landline, voice over Internet protocol (VoIP), and cellular networks.

The Federal Communications Commission also offers a free, 24/7/365 speech-to-speech service through a program called the Telecommunications Relay Service. The TRS allows people with hearing and speech disabilities to access the telephone system to place and receive calls.

Speech-to-speech lets people with a speech disability make telephone calls using their own voice (or an assistive voice device). Similar to all the other forms of TRS, an operator specially trained in understanding a variety of speech disorders will relay the conversation back and forth between the person with the speech disability and the other party. Dial the TRS center at 711 and indicate that you wish to make a speech-to-speech call.

Innovations in speech recognition are changing the game for augmented communicators and shattering myths that computers must sound robotic and monotonous. Today, AAC devices and

other assistive technologies can help people with speech disabilities gain greater independent access to leisure, learning, and
employment. The best place to start is with a speech/language
pathologist who has experience in augmentative and alternative
communication to help you select the right device.

There are so many factors involved—from motor skills to
language and cognitive abilities, vocabulary needs, and even the
design and style of the device. A friend of mine who uses an AAC
device once remarked to me, "I'm thirty-three years old. I don't
want pictures of bananas and apples on my computer screen."
Fortunately, he found exactly what he needed—a high-functioning,
word-based system. Knowing the factors involved should help you
figure out what you need, too.

Assistive Technology and the Americans With Disabilities Act

8

For most people technology makes things easier. For people with disabilities, however, technology makes things possible. In some cases, especially in the workplace, technology becomes the great equalizer and provides the person with a disability a level playing field on which to compete.

—Mary Radabaugh, former employee at IBM's
Disability Support Center

The Americans with Disabilities Act (ADA) extends full civil rights and equal opportunities to people with disabilities in both the public and private sectors. Specifically, the law prohibits discrimination in employment, public services, public accommodations, and telecommunications on the basis of a physical or mental disability. The ADA is modeled on the Rehabilitation Act of 1973, which prohibits discrimination in services and employment on the basis of handicap.

George H. W. Bush, the forty-first president of the United States, signed the Americans with Disabilities Act into law. It has three sections, or titles:

- Title I prohibits employment discrimination by private employers, state and local governments, employment agencies, and labor unions.
- Title II prohibits discrimination in all programs, activities, and services of public entities, including government agencies and public schools.
- Title III prohibits discrimination in places of public accommodation, such as restaurants, movie theaters, shopping centers, banks, and private schools.

Assistive technology helps realize the full potential of the ADA. Under the law, employers, state agencies, local governments, and other places of public accommodation may have a responsibility to provide assistive technology as "reasonable accommodations" and to make their services and programs otherwise accessible.

In the workplace, this isn't hard. Employers make accommodations for all of their employees. A chair, desk, computer, lighting, and safety equipment could all be considered accommodations that are made for all employees. In this sense, assistive technology is no different; it is simply any item that can assist an individual with a disability to succeed on the job.

The majority of assistive technology solutions are simple, inexpensive, low-tech devices such as a hands-free telephone or ergonomic keyboard.

Many of these accommodations are already in use in the workplace. For instance, a basic screen reader for the blind is built into both Windows and Mac computers. Speech-recognition software such as Dragon NaturallySpeaking is used by both busy CEOs and workers who are dyslexic. Instant messaging programs, free and used in offices everywhere, are also very useful for the deaf and hard or hearing.

Employers are required to provide "reasonable accommodations" such as assistive technology or a flexible work schedule if an employee (or a family member, health professional, or other representative) asks, provided fulfilling the request does not place an "undue burden" on the company. The requested technology must be acquired for a job-specific function; the employer is not required to purchase a personal device such as a hearing aid or wheelchair.

ADA Amendments Act

In March 2009 I interviewed an employment attorney for my Web site, Abledbody.com. Michael Soltis, managing partner of the Stamford, Conn., office of workplace law firm Jackson Lewis, told me that the ADA is now one of the top concerns for employers.

The ADA Amendments Act went into effect on January 1, 2009. The act broadened the definition of disability and overturned four Supreme Court rulings relating to the law. The ADA retains the original definition of disability as any physical or mental impairment that limits a "major life activity" but expands the list to include activities such as reading, bending, and communicating, as well as functions such as brain, respiratory, and reproductive functions.

The act also clarifies that an impairment that is episodic or in remission—such as epilepsy, diabetes, or cancer—is a disability if it would substantially limit a major life activity when active.

The effect of these changes is to make it easier for an individual seeking protection under the ADA to establish that he or she has a disability within the meaning of the ADA.

Amendments to the ADA have expanded disability protections but have also caused some confusion as to what constitutes a disability. Soltis says that employees and employers should engage in an "interactive dialogue" that will give employees with disabilities a method to make the strongest case possible for their accommodation needs, while steering companies away from fraudulent charges of discrimination and reckless lawsuits.

Making the Case for Accommodation

Q&A with Michael Soltis, Managing Partner, Jackson Lewis LLC.

Q: Mike, what's an interactive dialogue?

A: It's a process that helps the employer determine whether a reasonable accommodation is necessary, reasonable, and feasible to enable an employee to remain in his or her position. The court considers the interactive dialogue as one way in which the company can show its efforts to address the request for accommodation. At the same time, it helps the employee to strengthen his or her case for an accommodation because they're supplying the employer with relevant facts, such as a medical note, needed to assess the situation more acutely. That's why the whole dialogue should be documented, on both ends.

Q: How does an interactive dialogue work?

A: There's no set approach, but there are a few principles that have been established in court. One is that both employer and employee must dialogue appropriately. This is a good-faith issue that says both parties must work together in the search for a reasonable accommodation. It is the employee's job to educate the employer on what he needs, but the employee needs to be open-minded as well. He can't insist on a single, unreasonable accommodation. That would cause the breakdown of the interactive process.

Q: When does the accommodation discussion need to happen?

A: It's either triggered by the employee, who requests the accommodation, or by the employer, who recognizes the need to have the interactive dialogue. But an employee doesn't need to use any specific words when making a request. They should use plain English and need not mention the ADA or the phrase reasonable accommodation. What matters isn't the formality, rather that the employee provides the employer with enough information so that the employer can deduce both the disability and the desire for an accommodation. It's not even necessary for the worker to suggest certain remedies. This is up to the employer to figure out. But at the same time, the employer isn't a mind reader. There's a case where someone asked for an accommodation and then sued her employer for not providing the specific one she wanted. The other thing is that the request has to be timely. You can't wait until you're fired or caught sleeping on the job to ask for an accommodation. That's not an accommodation—that's a second chance in the court's eyes.

Q: How does an employer start the interactive dialogue?

A: There's a bit of homework involved at first. First, they should analyze the particular job involved and determine its purpose and essential functions. Second, they need to consult with the individual to ascertain the precise job-related limitations and how those limitations could be overcome with a reasonable accommodation. The third step is to work with the individual to identify potential accommodations and assess the effectiveness each would have. And fourth, consider the preference of the individual to be accommodated and select the accommodation that is most appropriate for both the employee and the employer.

Q: What if the dialogue doesn't lead to a reasonable accommodation?

A: Engaging in the dialogue does not mean that an accommodation exists. Sometimes, a disability cannot be accommodated without undue hardship. A company may be able to terminate a disabled employee after concluding that it cannot reasonably accommodate the individual, but they should make every effort possible, including looking into vacant positions elsewhere in the company for which the employee is qualified. Where no reasonable accommodation exists, however, an employer need not continue to engage in a futile dialogue.

Q: What happens if the interactive dialogue doesn't work and the employee sues their employer?

A: The court will look at the interactive process to determine whether there's evidence to show that one party's bad faith caused the breakdown in dialogue. The dialogue is a means to an end, the end being the identification of a reasonable accommodation. Generally, an employer who fails to dialogue appropriately violates the ADA only if a reasonable accommodation existed and they didn't seek it out or implement it. However, in some states, an employer's failure to engage in the interactive process is a per se violation of the state's antidiscrimination law, regardless of whether an accommodation exists.

Q: What's something an employee might not know about the interactive dialogue and the ADA?

A: During this time, an employer has the right to ask for relevant information, including a medical note from a doctor. The note doesn't have to discuss the specifics of the condition, just that the employee may need an accommodation for certain symptoms.

Though Title I of the ADA prohibits discrimination against the disabled, the unemployment numbers speak for themselves. In 2008, only 46 percent of working-age people with disabilities held jobs, compared with 84 percent of nondisabled people. The national unemployment rate for people with disabilities was 12.9 percent in April 2009, compared with 8.6 percent for nondisabled Americans.

The good news is that assistive technologies can—and will—level the playing field. Just like my tag line for Abledbody.com reads, assistive technology provides the "can-do, done differently" enabling devices that drive opportunities for people with disabilities across the board.

How to Pay for Assistive Technology 9

> *The cost of freedom is always high.*
> —John F. Kennedy

Finding and buying the appropriate assistive technology for your needs can be a daunting task. Not only do you need to assess critically which technologies you need; you also have to find a way to pay for them.

There's no centralized place for assistive technology funding. Often, people with disabilities depend on a myriad federal and state government programs and social benefits for assistive technology devices. But eligibility is difficult to establish in some cases. Other people look to private health insurance programs, but, again, criteria are stringent and the need must be rigorously defended.

There's a silver lining to this. According to the Job Accommodation Network (JAN), 80 percent of the accommodations that JAN suggests cost less than $500. The cost of assistive technology can be shared by the employer, the individual, and third-party payers such as employer-supported health insurance for the employee, workers' compensation, the state's department of rehabilitation services (also known as the department of vocational rehabilitation, or VocRehab), philanthropic organizations, and assistive technology loan programs.

However exorbitant the costs may seem at first, assistive technology doesn't have to break your bank account. There are many resources to help you get what you need or find alternatives to expensive equipment.

Employers and Educational Institutions

Under the ADA, employers, state agencies, local governments, and other places of public accommodations may have a responsibility to provide—and pay for—assistive technology for individuals as "reasonable accommodations and to otherwise make their services and programs accessible." K–12 school districts and postsecondary educational institutions that receive federal funds are included in this mandate.

For example, under the ADA an employer may be responsible for providing you with computer hardware and software that helps you perform job-specific functions such as reading documents or hearing on the telephone. Some companies, including Wal-Mart, allow for job aids for employees with conditions not currently recognized by law under the ADA.

Similarly, the Individuals with Disabilities Education Act (IDEA), a law that makes provisions for special needs children, includes assistive technology that facilitates classroom learning through what's called an individual education program, or IEP.

Note, however, that devices and gadgets become the property of the school or company when you leave.

Private Health Insurance

Private, group-based health insurance, such as the kind your employer provides to you and your family, is the best avenue for seeking assistive technology funding. Group insurance generally is offered through health maintenance organizations (HMOs) or preferred provider organizations (PPOs) that guarantee payment of medical expenses—including assistive technology medical equipment—in exchange for a monthly premium.

HMO and PPO plans differ from policy to policy, so check your policy regarding the qualifying criteria or contact your provider to find out whether your policy fully or partially covers assistive technology.

Private insurers usually have very strict eligibility requirements and caps on reimbursement. Nevertheless, depending on your policy, many devices such as wheelchairs and cochlear implants are covered under the durable medical equipment (DME), speech generating-device (SGD), or other categories. The company from which you're buying the device will be able to help you submit the appropriate paperwork and application to the insurer, but it's up to you to ascertain what the policy will and will not pay out.

Be sure to ask the insurance provider what information and documents they require up front, such as a doctor's note (and keep copies as they may get lost in the mail); the timeline for submitting and receiving a decision about your application; what deductions or monetary limitations, if any, apply to funding your assistive technology; and how the appeals process works if your application is denied.

If you are denied funding in the first round, double-check to see whether you have provided your insurance carrier with the required medical documentation and appropriate forms. If something has been completed incorrectly, the insurance company may not voluntarily notify you. Assuming everything was correct, you can ask for an administrative review by a staff physician or nurse.

Government Health Insurance

Medicare

This government program run by the Social Security Administration provides Americans aged sixty-five and older with health insurance. Medicare is also available to people with disabilities under the age of sixty-five, although they generally must already be receiving Social Security Disability Income (SSDI) or Supplemental Security Income (SSI) benefits.

Private insurance companies work with the Social Security Administration to provide Medicare insurance coverage, including paying for some medical equipment. If you pay into a separate plan called the Medicare Advantage plan, your Medicare benefits can be credited toward enrollment in an HMO or PPO, which offers better coverage of assistive technology equipment.

Medicaid

This federal and state health insurance program is for low-income individuals, though people with disabilities can qualify even if they don't meet the income requirements. It typically covers all medical needs but is more stringent about paying for assistive technology.

Veterans Affairs

If you're a veteran, the VA may purchase equipment for you. The type and amount of services available depend upon whether your disability was "service connected," meaning that it occurred or was aggravated during active duty. More services are available to veterans with service-connected disabilities.

Vocational Rehabilitation Agencies

Every state has a vocational rehabilitation agency that's supposed to fund equipment you need to keep a job or get an education. You have to provide proof that a certain device will enable you to enter or continue employment, live more independently, or improve your health.

You can get a list of state VocRehab agencies at www. disabilityinfo.gov.

Workers' Compensation

If you became disabled through a work-related accident, covering the cost of an assistive device may be the responsibility of workers' compensation insurance. When permanent disability is involved, workers' compensation carriers generally want to settle the claim as soon as possible. Do not settle the claim or sign any waivers or release forms until you have medical proof that the disability is permanent.

TIP *If one piece of equipment works better for you than another, document the superiority of the preferred device. Take notes and take photos. You may even want to make a video.*

Personal Loan

You may have to pay personally for a portion of the desired assistive technology. A personal bank loan or home equity loan may help you do so.

Under the Assistive Technology Act, the federal government provides grants to states to create financial loan programs that allow individuals with disabilities to purchase assistive technology at a lower-than-average interest rate. The Rehabilitation Engineering and Assistive Technology Society of North America (RESNA) Alternative Financing Technical Assistance Project (AFTAP) provides assistance to people seeking state financial loans.

Charitable Organizations

Search for a local civic or charitable organization, private foundation, or association in your area that can help raise the necessary funds.

Employer Tax Breaks

Tax credits and tax deductions may be available to employers who provide reasonable accommodations. The Internal Revenue Code allows a deduction of up to $15,000 per year for expenses associated with the removal of qualified architectural and transportation barriers.

Small businesses whose gross receipts are less than $1 million are eligible for a tax credit for certain costs of compliance with the ADA, including the costs of removing architectural, physical, communications, and transportation barriers; providing readers, interpreters, and other auxiliary aids; and acquiring or modifying equipment or devices.

Despite the obstacles, do not give up. Investigate and exhaust all possible funding avenues and alternatives. You may need to challenge some decisions in the process. Standing up for yourself and your rights is one of the demands of having a disability, but it makes you a stronger person in the long run.

The Future
of Assistive
Technology

10

I've often argued that people with physical disabilities who use assistive technology are functionally more "interesting" human beings because they've incorporated machines into their brains and bodies. In the 2008 movie *Iron Man*, the superhero escapes from a cave in Afghanistan in part by building a pair of robotic legs. This sci-fi movie is more grounded in reality than it might seem.

In 2008, researchers at a university in Japan unveiled a robotic suit that helps disabled people walk. The computerized suit, known as HAL (short for "hybrid assistive limb"), has sensors that read brain signals through the skin to direct limb movement. It's currently being produced by a Japanese company and will cost around $20,000. The invention of HAL will have far-reaching benefits for the disabled as well as the elderly, giving them the "potential to lift up to ten times the weight they normally could."

Other researchers around the world, including those at MIT, are working on similar robotic suits that increase mobility and lighten the burden for soldiers and others who carry heavy packs and equipment.

Robotics is also making its way into transportation. As cars for the masses evolve, so will the vehicles used by people with disabilities. There are now hydrogen-fueled wheelchairs and wheelchairs that let people stand up. Now car manufacturers are tinkering with personal mobility vehicles, which could also help people who use electronic wheelchairs or scooters.

GM and Segway have teamed up to create a two-wheeled, thirty-five-mile-per-hour vehicle called the PUMA (for "personal urban mobility and accessibility"). Toyota, too, is working on its personal mobility concept, called the i-unit. Both vehicles support autopilot and traffic-tracking mechanisms to help avoid accidents. A personalized recognition system can provide information and music. In the world of personal mobility, Hungarian company Rehab takes the cake. Its concept, dubbed the Kenguru, is specifically designed for wheelchair users. Starting from behind the car, the driver simply rolls into place, locks down the wheelchair, and drives off using a joystick controller. Futurists believe cars will someday be driverless, using a system of sensors.

Robotics is just one way that technology is changing the future for people with disabilities. Scientists around the world are also developing bionics, or products that combine natural and synthetic elements to create a more powerful technology.

In medicine, bionics means the replacement or enhancement of organs or other body parts with mechanical versions. The term became famous in the 1970s with the TV show *The Six Million Dollar Man*, in which a fictional astronaut was able to replace his legs, arm, and eye with "bionic" implants.

Today, thousands of people are recipients of bionic products. These devices, powered by microchips and miniature computer systems, are embedded in the human body and send neural signals from the disabled part of the body to the brain.

The most widely used bionic device today is the cochlear implant, which provides artificial hearing to people who are deaf. Cochlear implants work by implanting electrodes that replicate the damaged cells in the ear, enabling sound to be passed on to the brain. Researchers are also perfecting a bionic ear that would boost the growth of nerve cells in the inner ear when zapped with electricity.

Bionic eyes are an even newer technology. A firm called Optobionics has already begun implanting silicon microchips into the eye. The Optobionics device is made up of 5,000 microscopic light detectors that directly activate nerve cells in the eye, allowing electrical impulses to be sent to the brain and interpreted.

Another product in development is an artificial vision system that's installed in eyeglasses and enables the blind to see objects and faces. This system, which consists of a subminiature camera and an ultrasonic distance sensor, can record the visual world and transmit it directly to a person's brain.

Now for the brain. A new technology that has already been tested on a few patients is BrainGate, a brain implant that's designed to help those who have lost control of their limbs or other bodily functions, such as patients with amyotrophic lateral sclerosis or spinal cord injury. The implanted computer chip monitors brain activity in the patient and converts the intention of the user into computer commands.

Another burgeoning field is neural prosthetics, where the brain controls the prosthetic device. This will also help people who are paralyzed. University of Pittsburgh researchers are developing the first brain-controlled arm and hand that performs, looks, and feels like a real limb.

Today's prostheses are becoming more computer-like while more closely resembling human limbs. The i-LIMB Hand from Touch Bionics is a prosthetic hand with five individually powered fingers that looks and acts like a real human hand. The company also has a full-arm system in development.

Computer technology is constantly evolving, too, which will benefit people with disabilities. At the 2009 Assistive Technology Industry Association conference, I heard from a group called Raising the Floor, which hopes to bring the Internet to each and every person in the world, regardless of economic situation or disability. Under this scenario, a boy in Africa who is blind might access the Internet via a cell phone with a screen reader that he has set up as part of his personalized, Internet-based user profile.

The next frontier in computer technology is the talking computer, which has already begun with speech-recognition programs that use high-end voice synthesis. These programs still require users to train their computer to understand their voice, but in the near future we will see automatic speech recognition that can translate anyone's speech, in any language, into real-time text, offering promise to millions of deaf and hard-of-hearing individuals who still struggle to communicate over the phone and in noisy environments.

A conversation with Dan Hubbell, technical evangelist for Microsoft's Accessibility Business Unit

Q: What trends in assistive technology will we see over the next ten years?

A: Two key trends I am seeing are increased customization and increased portability of assistive technology. Consumers, especially those with disabilities, have a much greater need for flexibility in how they interact with computers and technology. More and more, computers will adjust to a person and the environment dynamically rather than requiring a person to adjust to how they use the computer like they do today. And with the continued miniaturization of technology it is increasingly possible to carry many of these tools with you. Our hope is to see technology that is flexible and portable enough to be accessed by anyone, anywhere, no matter what their abilities are.

Q: What's an example?

A: We are currently seeing a number of portable products coming to market like software that works on a GPS-enabled cell phone that can speak walking directions for a person with a visual disability.

Q: What about advances in newer assistive technologies, such as speech recognition?

A: Speech recognition for years has been becoming more mainstream and is increasingly integrated into computers and consumer electronics. But speech is just one of many new ways for consumers to use and interact with technology. Advances in touch, gesture, and optical tracking will allow users to use computers in a way that is most natural to them. Say you're typing a document in Microsoft Word and you decide you want to switch the order of two paragraphs. You reach up to the screen and highlight the first paragraph with your finger and move it to where you want it to appear in the document. Then you give the computer a spoken command to print the document. Having these various options are critical to success for people with disabilities in the workplace.

Q: Will we see any improvements in accessibility for products used in the home, such as washing machines?

A: Appliances that once were usable by most people have become increasingly inaccessible to people with disabilities. Manufacturers of copiers, microwave ovens, and washers and dryers, to name a few, have replaced physical push buttons and dials with touch screens and flat panel buttons for operation. These are designed to improve the user experience, but people who are blind or mobility impaired can't use them. New technology advances in home and office appliances— including microwave ovens, copiers, VCRs, thermostats, ATM machines, or kiosks—will make it possible to operate them remotely. The remote controlling device could be a personal computer, laptop, cell phone, or other mobile device that will be able to communicate remotely to manage and operate a variety of home and office appliances.

Q: What's one technology that you're most excited about?

A: I am excited to see that eventually more accessibility devices will be integrated to work with mobile technology like GPS, radio frequency identification (RFID), text-to-speech, and even Tag technology. These mobile devices might be woven into clothing, worn in the ear, attached to a wheelchair, or even become a new form of fashion jewelry. They will not only be able to manipulate our environment by turning lights on or off, or adjusting a thermostat, but they will also inform us of where we are and provide critical information about our environment. This will put everyone in control and allow them to interact and manipulate their environment, regardless of ability, through the method of their choice. The next generation of technology will be life changing for everyone, but especially for people with disabilities. When an employee who is blind can easily navigate through a new office building with no assistance other than the computer he always carries with him as a lapel pin, we'll know the future has arrived.

Speech-recognition development offers the most direct line from the computers of today to true artificial intelligence. Heard of the Turing test? In 1951 British mathematician Alan Turing proposed a test of a machine's ability to demonstrate intelligence. When technology gets to a point where a human cannot tell whether he or she is speaking to a computer or another human, the machine will have passed the Turing test. Raymond Kurzweil, who developed the first large-vocabulary speech-recognition program, has predicted that we will see Turing test–capable computers in 2029.

And one more for *Star Trek* fans: next-generation technology will include three-dimensional holograms that can beam video into homes, offices, and hospitals. Think of the benefits for people who are deaf and need an instant sign-language interpreter, or for someone with an intellectual disability who needs a caregiver's instructions or attention.

At the heart of the future of assistive technology lies universal and accessible design. This is the philosophy that states that technology should be created from the ground up with the needs of everyone in mind, including people with disabilities. While we're not quite there, more companies are considering the cost advantages of not having to retrofit their products to meet the needs of differently abled people.

Today we're seeing more homes being built more "universally" to allow people to stay in their homes as they age or become disabled. Another trend is to build smart homes, where various technologies and appliances communicate with each other through a local network. This helps people with disabilities stay in their homes and maintain their independence and safety, while letting caregivers monitor their activities from remote locations. The monitoring or safety devices that can be installed in a home include lighting and motion sensors, environmental controls (which I discussed in chapter 5), video cameras, automatic timers for food and medicine reminders, emergency assistance programs, and alerts, such as detecting when the oven has been left on by accident.

The future looks brighter every day for assistive technologies, thanks to the commitment of scientists, doctors, and researchers who make it their mission to help people with disabilities. We must also offer thanks to the educators who take the time to find different ways for children to learn, and to companies that work hard to make their offices accessible and their people diverse. And to families, friends, and caregivers everywhere, who are with us every step of the way as we navigate these new technologies (and sometime test them out on them).

Throughout this book I've explored the concept of "can-do, done differently," a concept I truly believe in. People with disabilities can do anything anyone without a disability can do, just differently. In order to maximize our potential through technology, we must first recognize our abilities. More than anything, it is how we arm ourselves with knowledge and maintain a positive attitude that makes the difference. Remember: in every body there is more potential with the help of assistive technology. Now that you have all the enabling technologies you need, go out there and live your life to the fullest.

|Resources

You can learn more about the products mentioned in this book by going to the Web sites of the assistive technology companies who manufacture and sell them. Many have detailed product descriptions, pricing information, videos, online demos and tutorials, and free trial downloads of their software. The vendors mentioned in this book include the following:

ALL DISABILITIES

Apple
1 Infinite Loop
Cupertino, CA 95014
1-800-676-2775
www.apple.com

Mac and iPhone

Microsoft
1 Microsoft Way
Redmond, WA 98052
1-800-Microsoft
www.microsoft.com

PC and Windows Mobile Phones

COGNITIVE

Ablelink Technologies
618 N. Nevada Ave.
Colorado Springs, CO 80903
1-719-592-0347
ablelinktech.com

Pocket Coach

AssistiveWare
Amsterdam
31-20-6128266
www.assistiveware.com
info@assistiveware.com

Proloquo2go

Cambium Learning
313 Spleen Street
Natick, MA 01760
1-800-547-6747
www.cambiumlearning.com
info@cambiumlearning.com

Intellikeys

Don Johnston
26799 West Commerce Drive
Volo, IL 60073
1-800-999-4660
www.donjohnston.com
info@donjohnston.com

Write Out Loud

Livescribe
7677 Oakport St. 12th Floor
Oakland, CA 94621
1–877–727–4239
www.livescribe.com
info@livescribe.com

Livescribe Pulse Pen

Premier Assistive Technology
1309 N. William St.
Joliet, IL 60435
1-815-927-7390
www.premierathome.com

Various Products

Texthelp Systems Inc.
100 Unicorn Park Drive
Woburn, MA 01801
1-888-248-0652
www.texthelp.com
u.s.info@texthelp.com

Software

WizCom Technologies
234 Littleton Road
Westford, MA 01886
1-888-777-0552
www.wizcomtech.com
usa.info@wizcomtech.com

Various Products

COMMUNICATION

AbleNet Inc.
2808 Fairview Avenue North
Roseville, MN 55113
1-800-322-0956
www.ablenetinc.com
customerservice@ablenetinc.com

SuperTalker

Access Ingenuity
3635 Montgomery Drive
Santa Rosa, CA 95405
1-877-579-4380
www.accessingenuity.com

Various products

ArtefactSoft Inc.
12361 Brown Fox Way
Reston, VA 20191
1-703-869-1479
www.artefactsoft.com
info@artefactsoft.com

DAF/FAF Assistant

Casa Futura Technologies
720 31st Street
Boulder, CO 80303
1-888-FLU-ENCY
www.casafuturatech.com
sales@casafuturatech.com

SmallTalk Fluency Device

Dynavox Mayer-Johnson
2100 Wharton Street
Pittsburgh, PA 15203
1-866-396-2869
www.dynavox.com

Boardmaker, V/Vmax

**The Great Talking Box
Company**
2528 Qume Dr.
San Jose, CA 95131
1-877-275-4482
www.greattalkingbox.com

Easy Talk

Gus Communications
1006 Lonetree Court
Bellingham, WA 98229
1-866-487-1006
www.gusinc.com
admin@gusinc.com

Various Products

Janus Development Group
112 Staton Road
Greenville, NC 27834
1-866-551-9042
www.janusdevelopment.com
customerserv@janusdevelopment.com

SpeechEasy Fluency Device

JITA Technologies
4905 Mission Street
San Francisco, CA 94112
1-800-661-9048
http://buyersguide.asha.org
inof@jitatech.com

Speech Assistant

Sonic Alert
1081 West Innovation Dr.
Kearney, MO 64060
1-816-628-1949
www.teltex.com
info@teltex.com

Sonic Boom Alarm Clock

HEARING

Able Planet Inc.
9500 W. 49th Ave.
Wheat Ridge, CO 80033
1-877-266-1979
www.ableplanet.com
info@ableplanet.com

Noise-cancelling Headphones

Advanced Bionics
25129 Rye Canyon Loop
Valencia, CA 91355
1-877-829-0026
www.advancedbionics.com
hear@advancedbionics.com

Cochlear Implant

Audex
710 Standard Street
Longview, TX 75604
1-800-237-0716
www.audex.com
paula@audex.com

Cordless Amplified Phone

Bellman & Symfon
Sweden
+46 (0) 31-682820
www.bellman.com
info@bellman.se

Bellman Visit

Clarity
4289 Bonny Oaks Drive
Chattanooga, TN 37406
1-800-426-3738
www.clarityproducts.com

Various Hearing Products

ClearSounds
8160 S. Madison Street
Burr Ridge, IL 60527
1-800-965-9043
www.clearsounds.com

Neckloop, Amplified Phone

Comlink
1900 Annapolis Lane
Plymouth, MN 55441
1-763-557-6434
www.comlinkproducts.com
info@comlinkproducts.com

Personal Sound Enhancer

**Communication Service for
the Deaf**
102 North Krohn Place
Sioux Falls, SD 57103
1-605-367-5760
www.c-s-d.org

Relay

Global Assistive Devices
1121 East Commercial Boulevard
Oakland Park, FL 33334
1-954-776-1373
www.globalassistive.peachhost.com
info@globalassistive.com

Handset Amplifier

Hamilton Relay Services
1006 12th St
Aurora, NE 68818
1-402-694-5299
www.hamiltonnationalrelay.com

Relay

Harris Communications
15155 Technology Drive
Eden Prairie, MN 55344
1-800-843-3544
www.harriscomm.com
info@harriscomm.com

Various Hearing Products

iCommunicator
Brooklyn, NY
1-718-965-8600
www.myicommunicator.com
icomm-support@myicommunicator.com

Software

Media Access Group WGBH
1 Guest Street
Boston, MA 02135
1-617-300-3600
http://main.wgbh.org
access@wgbh.org

Various Services

Oticon
Denmark
45-39-177100
www.oticon.com
contact-us@oticon.com

Streamer

Phonak
Switzerland
41-58-9280101
www.phonak.com
contact@phonak.ch

Icom

Purple Communications
773 San Marin Drive
Novato, CA 94945
1-877-885-3172
www.purple.us
support@purple.us

Relay, Netbook

QualiLife SA
Riva Paradiso 26
Paradiso, Switzerland
++41 (0) 91 980.09.51
www.qualilife.com
info@qualilife.com

Software

**Rochester Institute of
Technology (C-Print)**
52 Lomb Memorial Drive
Rochester, NY 14623
1-585-475-7557 (Voice/TTY)
http://cprint.rit.edu

C-print

Sensorcom
London, UK
BR3 4LZ 44 (0) 870-901-6070
www.sensorcom.com
info@sensorcom.com

T-Link

Sorenson Communications
4192 South Riverboat Road
Salt Lake City, UT 84123
1-866-877-9826
www.sorenson.com

Videophone, Relay Service

TecEar
30215 Woodgate Drive
Southfield, MI 48076
1-248-867-2759
www.tecear.com
info@tecear.com

Various Hearing Products

ULTECH
65 Fern Street c/o Mark Hall
Waterbury, CT 06704
1-203-574-5128
www.mhsa.us

Caption Mic

Ultratec
450 Science Drive
Madison, WI 53711
1-888-269-7477
www.captionedtelephone.com
captel@captelmail.com

Captel; TTY

Vivid Acoustics (Inclusion Solutions)
6909 N. Western Ave.
Chicago, IL 60645
1-773-338-9612
www.inclusionsolutions.com
contact@inclusionsolutions.com

Hearing Loops

Williams Sound
10321 W. 70th Street
Eden Prairie, MN 55344
1-800-328-6190
www.williamssound.com
info@williamssound.com

Bellman Audio Maxi, Pocketalker

PHYSICAL

Broadened Horizons' Gimp Gear
15382 80th Place North
Maple Grove, MN 55311
1-877-6-GIMPGEAR
www.gimpgear.com

Various Products

Hunter Digital
7310 W. 82nd St.
Los Angeles, CA 90045
1-800-57 MOUSE
www.footmouse.com
support@footmouse.com

NoHands Mouse

Independent Tools
1281 E. Magnolia
Fort Collins, CO 80524
1-970-223-0425
www.pocketdresser.com

Pocket Dresser

Infogrip
1794 East Main Street
Ventura, CA 93001
1-805-652-0770
www.infogrip.com
info@infogrip.com

BIG Track Mouse

LC Technologies
3919 Old Lee Highway Suite 81B
Fairfax, VA 22030
1-866-603-2195
www.eyegaze.com
info0309@eyegaze.com

Eyegaze Edge

Levo U.S.A.
7105 Northland Terrace
Brooklyn Park, MN 55428
1-888-LEVOUSA
www.levousa.com
teamlevousa@danetechnologies.com

Wheelchair

Madentec
4664 99 Street
Edmonton, Canada T6E 5H5
1-877-623-3682
www.madentec.com
info@madentec.com

Various Products

Origin Instruments
845 Greenview Drive
Grand Prairie, TX 75050
1-888-656-6141
www.orin.com
support@orin.com

Mouse

Prentke Romich Co.
1022 Heyl Road
Wooster, OH 44691
1-800-262-1984
www.prentrom.com
info@prentrom.com

ECO and ECOPoint

RJ Cooper & Associates
27601 Forbes Rd.
Laguna Niguel, CA 92677
1-949-582-2572
www.rjcooper.com
info@rjcooper.com

Mini Auggie, Super Auggie

SAJE Technology
765 Dixon Court
Hoffman Estates, IL 60190
1-847-756-7603
www.saje-tech.com

Various Products

Sunrise Medical
3443 E. Central Ave
Fresno, CA 94650
1-866-391-9911
www.sunrisemedical.com
webmaster@sunmed.com

Wheelchair

Touch Bionics
2 Edgewater Drive
Middletown, NY 10940
1-845-343-4668
www.touchbionics.com
info@touchbionics.com

iLIMB

TRAXSYS
East Portway
Andover, UK SP10 3LU
44 (0) 1264-349-640
www.traxsys.com
sales@traxsys.com

Joystick

Toyota
19001 South Western Ave. Dept.
WC11
Torrance, CA 90501
1-800-331-4331
www.toyota.com

Sienna

**Wacom Technology
Corporation**
1311 SE Cardinal Court
Vancouver, WA 98683
1-800-922-6613
www.wacom.com

Bamboo Tablet

Words+
40015 Sierra Highway, Building
B-145
Palmdale, CA 93550
1-800-869-8521
www.words-plus.com
info@words-plus.com

FreedomLITE

7020 AC Skinner Pkwy, Suite 100
Jacksonville, FL 32256
1-877-TEAM-WWP
www.woundedwarriorproject.org

Wounded Warrior Project

VISION

ABISee
77 PowderMill Road
Acton, MA 01720
1-800-681-5909
www.abisee.com
info@abisee.com

Zoomex, Solo

Amazon
1200 12th Avenue South Suite 1200
Seattle, WA 98144
1-866-216-1072
www.amazon.com

Kindle

**American Printing House for
the Blind**
1839 Frankfort Avenue
Louisville, KY 40206
1-800-223-1839
www.aph.org
info@aph.org

Various Products

Bookshare (Benetech Initiative)
480 California Ave.
Palo Alto, CA 94306
1-650-475-5440
www.bookshare.org
info@benetech.org

Bookshare.org

Brytech
2301 St. Laurent Blvd.
Ottawa, ON K1G 4J7
1-800-263-4095
www.brytech.com
inquiries@brytech.com

Note Teller

Code Factory
Spain
34-937-337-66
www.codefactory.es

Mobile Magnifier, GEO

Dell
One Dell Way
Round Rock, TX 78664
1-800-624-9896
www.dell.com

Inspiron Mini

En-vision America
1845 West Hovey Avenue
Normal, IL 61761
1-800-890-1180
www.envisionamerica.com

ID Mate

Freedom Scientific
11800 31st Court North
St. Petersburg, FL 33716
1-877-775-9474
www.freedomscientific.com

Topaz, JAWS, PACMate

GW Micro
725 Airport North Office Park
Fort Wayne, IN 46825
1-866-339-1180
www.gwmicro.com
sales@gwmicro.com

Windows Eyes, Braille Sense

HumanWare
445 Parc Industriel
Longueil, Canada J4H 3V7
1-800-722-3393
www.humanware.com
ca.info@humanware.com

Smartview Extend; My Reader;
  Braille Note, Victor Stream

knfb Reading Technology
P.O. Box 620128
Newton Lower Falls, MA 02462
1-866-548-7323
www.knfbreader.com
Lisa@knfbReader.com

knfbReader and
  knfbReader Mobile

**Kurzweil Educational
Systems**
14 Crosby Drive #302
Bedford, MA 01730
1-800-894-5374
www.kurzweiledu.com
info@kurzweiledu.com

Kurzweil 3000

Maxi Aids
42 Executive Blvd.
Farmingdale, NY 11735
1-800-522-6294
www.maxiaids.com

Various Products

Nuance Communications
1 Wayside Road
Burlington, MA 01803
1-888-634-8200
www.nuance.com

Zoom, Dragon Nat'lly Speaking

**NV Access (NVDA
Screenreader)**
www.nvda-project.org

Nonvisual Desktop Access
  Screen Reader

Optelec
3030 Enterprise Court
Vista, CA 92081
1-800-826-4200
www.optelec.com
info@optelec.com

Farview Magnifier

Perkins School for the Blind
175 North Beacon Street
Watertown, MA 02472
1-617-924-3434
www.perkins.org
info@perkins.org

Brailler

Permobil
6961 Eastgate Blvd.
Lebanon, TN 37090
1-800-736-0925
www.permobil.com/USA
info@permobil.com

Wheelchair

Plextor
5737 Mesmer Ave
Culver City, CA 90230
1-877-792-4768
www.plextalk.com

Plextalk Pocket

Renaissance Learning
2911 Peach St.
Wisconsin Rapids, WI 54494
1-800-338-4204
www.renlearn.com

NEO Alphasmart and DANA WP

Sensory Software
4a Court Road
Malvern, UK
WR14 3BL 01684 578868
www.sensorysoftware.com
info@sensorysoftware.com

The Grid

Serotek Group
1128 Harmon Place Suite 310
Minneapolis, MN 55403
www.serotek.com

System Access Screen Reader

Shoplowvision.com
(JP Eyewear)
3030 Enterprise Court
Vista, CA 92081
1-800-826-4200
www.shoplowvision.com
ahardy@shoplowvision.com

Eyewear

There are many organizations that can assist you with finding assistive technology:

ABLEDATA is a database of information on assistive technology and rehabilitation equipment available in the United States. Funded by the National Institute on Disability and Rehabilitation Research, it contains more than 29,000 product listings and covers everything from white canes and adaptive clothing to low-vision reading systems and voice output programs.

www.abledata.com

The Alliance for Technology Access (ATA) is a national network of technology resource centers, organizations, individuals, and companies.

www.ataaccess.org

The Assistive Technology Industry Association is a not-for-profit membership organization of manufacturers, sellers, and providers of technology-based assistive devices and services.

www.atia.org

Assistivetech.net is an online information resource created by Georgia Tech's Center for Assistive Technology and Environmental Access, under funding from the National Institute on Disability and Rehabilitation Research. It provides information on assistive technologies and related resources.

www.assistivetech.net

DisabilityInfo.gov provides information about disability programs, services, laws, and benefits in your state.

www.disabilityinfo.gov

The Job Accommodation Network is a service of the U.S. Department of Labor's Office of Disability Employment Policy. It is an information and consulting service run by the International Center for Disability Information at West Virginia University and provides a free, comprehensive online database of job accommodations available, categorized by disability and job function. JAN also provides information regarding the Americans with Disabilities Act and other legislation.

www.jan.wvu.edu

The Rehabilitation Engineering and Assistive Technology Society of North America (RESNA) is an association for the advancement of rehabilitation and assistive technology. It promotes research and development, education, advocacy, and provision of technology and supports people with disabilities and others who are engaged in these activities.

www.resna.org

Index